The Great American Food Fight

WINNING THE BATTLE FOR FAMILY HEALTH

DR. BRENT BALDASARE

10 9 8 7 6 5 4 3 2 1

Copyright © 2016 by Brent Baldasare

Library of Congress Control Number: 2015960060

ISBN 978-0-983-24316-8

Dedication

This book is dedicated to my family: To my mother and sisters, who have always supported me. To my children, Lyndsey, Braxton and Makenna, whose healthy future is worth fighting for. To my wife, Angela, who titled this book and sustains me in everything, always. To my editor, relentless researcher, and mother-in-law, Dr. Cynthia Rogers Parks. And to my patient family, past, present and future.

Disclaimer

This book presents the research and ideas of the authors. It is not intended to be a substitute for personal consultation with nutritional or medical professionals and is not for the purpose of diagnosing, treating, curing or preventing any disease. Use of commercial and trade names does not imply approval or constitute endorsement, nor is criticism implied of any products not mentioned. The authors and the publisher do not assume any liability for ways in which the information present in the text is applied or interpreted, or for any loss, damage or injury incurred by relying on the information contained herein.

Contents

Foreword xiii

Preface.. xvii

Chapter 1. The Battle of Our Lives............................21

Fatter, Sicker, Dying Younger 23

Diabetes...24

Cardiovascular Disease 25

Cancer 25

Other Illnesses...26

Choosing to Be Fat and Sick? 27

Narrowing Food Choice.......................................28

Subsidizing Death and Disease 30

Promoting Death and Disease 32

Disguising Death and Disease 35

Engineering Death and Disease 36

Fighting Back 37

Eating in the Meantime..40

Chapter 2. All the Pretty Packages: 43

Buyer Beware..43

Getting Past the Package......................................43

Packaging Sneaks and Cheats 45

Packaging to Price...45

Black Hole Tactics 46

Front-of-Pack Labeling 48

Product Identification.......................................49

Statement of Identity 49

Health Claims..50

Qualified and Unqualified Health Claims.................51

Structure/Function Claims 52

Consumer Confusion over Health Claims 52

Product Endorsements...53

Ecology and Ethics Labels 54

Country of Origin Labels 55

Expiration Dates..55

Pictures and Graphics.......................................56

Poison Packaging 56

    BPA...57

    DEHP 59

Plastic Coding 60

Eating in the Meantime......................................61

Chapter 3. Bragging Up Front:

Nutrition Claims on Packaging...........................65

    Who Decides What's Healthy? 65

        The Nutritional Standards Alphabet 66

        Core Nutrient Content Claims 67

    Enriched and Fortified Claims 68

        Functional Foods......................................69

        Calorie Claims 70

        Carbohydrate Claims 71

        Cholesterol Claims...................................71

        Fat Claims 72

        Fiber Claims..73

        Freshness Claims 73

        Grain Claims 74

        Natural Claims 74

        Organic Claims 75

        Salt Claims...77

        Sugar Claims..78

    Dietary Guidance Symbols 79

    Shelf-Tag Labels 80

    The Future of Food Labeling 81

Eating in the Meantime......................................82

Chapter 4. Food Additives:

Subtracting from your Family's Health 85

    Who's Minding the Chemical Store?...................87

    How Do We Know It's Safe?............................89

Additives under Suspicion 90
  Azodicarbonamide 90
  Benzoic Acid, Sodium Benzoate 91
  Butylated Hydroxyanisole (BHA) 91
  Butylated Hydroxytoluene (BHT) 92
  Calcium Propionate...92
  Carrageenan 92
  Diacetyl 94
  Disodium Guanylate 95
  Monosodium Glutamate (MSG) 95
  MSG in Disguise...96
  Potassium Bromate 96
  Propyl Gallate 97
  Sulfites 97
Food Color Additives..98
  Color Additive Health Risks......................................99
  Identifying Color Additives 101
  Insect-based Colors..101
Progress on Color Additives 102
Eating in the Meantime..103

Chapter 5. The Big Fat Lies about Fat..........................105
The Big Fat Lie about Heart Disease 106
The Big Fat House of Cards...108
The Role of Fat...110
Types of Fat 111
  Saturated Fats...111
  Monounsaturated Fats...112
  Polyunsaturated Fats 112
Essential Fatty Acids: Omegas 3, 6, and 9...................113
  Trans Fats and Hydrogenation 114
Solid Cooking Fats...115
  Lard..115
  Shortening 115
  Butter..116

Margarine 117

Cooking Oils 118

Fake Fats 124

Eating in the Meantime 126

Chapter 6. Meaty Problems..........................129

Drugging Our Meat 130

Antibiotics..130

Ractopamine 132

Steroids and Growth Hormones.................133

Meat Fillers and Extenders.........................134

Pink Slime..135

Cellulose, Meat Glue, and More 136

Salt Water...137

Grass Fed vs. Corn Fed 137

Meat and Mortality.....................................138

Hot Dogs and Other Processed Meat 139

Nitrates and Nitrites 139

Chicken and Poultry....................................141

Organic Poultry 142

Free Range and Cage Free 142

Fish and Seafood 143

PCBs 143

Mercury...143

No Organic Fish 144

Genetically Modified Fish 145

Meat Substitutes..145

In vitro meat 145

Mycoprotein 146

Ethical and Environmental Issues 147

What about Protein? 148

Eating in the Meantime 149

Chapter 7. Milking the Public:
What's in the Dairy Case? 151

The Perfect Food? 151

   Osteoporosis...152

   The Skinny on Milk and Weight Loss 153

GMO Milk...154

   Cancer 156

   Early Puberty 157

   Acne 158

   Allergies...158

   Lactose Intolerance 159

   Parkinson's..159

The Raw Milk War..160

   Doing a Body No Good 161

   Consumers Speaking Out.......................................162

Non Dairy Milks 162

   Almond Milk..162

   Coconut Milk 163

   Rice Milk 163

   Soy Milk...163

   Dried and Powdered Milk 164

Cultured Dairy Foods..164

   Cheese 164

   Yogurt 165

Butter..165

Eggs...166

   Organic vs. Non-organic Eggs 166

   Animal Care Certified Eggs...................................167

   Omega-3 Eggs...168

   Brown vs. White 169

   Processed Eggs, Egg Substitutes...........................169

Eating in the Meantime 169

Chapter 8. Genetically Modified Food 171

No Scientific Consensus 173

Promises Unfulfilled 174

   GM Crops Will Increase Yields..............................174

GMO Crops Require Fewer Pesticides 175

GM Crops Are Better for the Environment 176

    Water 176

    Biodiversity 177

    Soil 178

GM will Keep Food Prices Low 179

GMOs Will Solve Food Scarcity 181

A Better Way 182

A Global Awakening 183

The U.S. Battle for Labeling 184

    What's in the Pipeline 185

    What's at Stake 186

Eating in the Meantime 187

Chapter 9. Produce and Poisons 191

The Pesticide Treadmill 193

Pesticide-Induced Diseases 194

    ADHD, Learning Disabilities 195

    Autism 195

    Birth/Fetal Effects 195

    Cancer 196

    Parkinson's 197

    Reproductive Dysfunction 197

    Obesity and Diabetes 198

Kids and Pesticides 198

    Pesticides and Wildlife 199

    Regulating Pesticides 200

Eating Pesticides 201

    The Dirty Dozen and Clean Fifteen 201

    Is Organic Worth the Price? 201

    Is Organic Food Pesticide Free? 203

Eating in the Meantime 204

Chapter 10. The Sour Truth about Sugar
and Artificial Sweeteners 207

Too Much of a Sweet Thing 207
Sugar and Disease 208
   Insulin Resistance 209
   Leptin Resistance 210
   It's the Sugar. *Really.* 210
Sugar Addiction 212
Knowing Our Sugars 213
Nutritive Sweeteners 213
   Sucrose 213
   Fructose 213
   High-Fructose Corn Syrup 214
   Sugar Alcohols 215
Non-Nutritive Sweeteners 215
   Aspartame 215
   Acesulfame K 217
   Saccharin 217
   Sucralose 218
   Neotame 219
   Rebiana 220
   Stevia 221
   Tagatose 221
Artificial Sugars and Weight Gain 222
Eating in the Meantime 223

Chapter 11. Dangers in Our Daily Bread 225
What's Happened to Wheat? 226
Wheat and Disease 227
Gluten-Related Disorders 227
   Celiac Disease 227
   Dermatitis Herpetiformis 228
   Gluten Sensitivity 228
   Wheat allergy 229
Gluten-Free Labeling 229
The Downsides of Gluten Free 229
Hidden Gluten 230

Eating in the Meantime 231

Chapter 12. The Fight For Real Food 233
  The Fight for Organic Food 233
  The Fight for Local Food 235
  and Community Agriculture 235
  The Fight for Real School Food.................................237
  The Fight for Food Transparency 240
Eating in the Meantime 241

Appendix...245
  BPA Free Products...245
  Colorings and Dyes..247
  Cooking with Fats and Oils.......................................249
  Smoke Points of Fats and Oils 250
  Safe Minimum Cooking Temperatures.......................251
  Types of Food Ingredients 252
  MSG Substitutes 255
  Plastic Coding 256
  Non-Dairy Sources of Calcium..................................258
  Non-Meat Sources of Protein....................................260
  Hidden Sugars 265
  Natural Sweeteners...266
  Sources of Gluten...268
References...270
Index 283

Foreword

By
Ocean Robbins

The human species, it's fair to say, has always been engaged in a food fight. Throughout most of our history, however, that battle was a pretty basic one—securing enough calories to survive. Even the advent of agriculture, a relatively recent phenomenon, didn't guarantee a dependable harvest or certain survival.

Only in this last century, with the introduction of large-scale industrial farming, global transportation systems, and the technological and scientific developments that have allowed for production and preservation, has the focus of food enlarged to include much more than mere subsistence. Modern supermarkets may stock more than 500 different kinds of breakfast cereals—far more than anyone could possibly need for mere survival. We can now choose among Chinese, Italian, Thai, Mexican, or Middle Eastern foods, all without having to leave our home town. We have a stunning array of flavors, textures and styles to choose from in foodstuffs, and most of us can access food grown 6,000 miles away, and processed 2,000 miles away, at our local store. Food is varied, abundant and accessible and, when measured as a fraction of disposable income, cheaper than it's ever been in human history.

As we're learning, however, the rapid changes that have brought us lots of cheap food have actually come with a terrible cost. We're paying a lot for that abundant, cheap food.

We're paying in the loss of natural resources, in the degradation of our planet's ecosystems, and in the rising rates of diet-related chronic disease. A price is being paid by the animals whose lives are subject to unspeakable cruelty, and by the farm workers who are exposed to so many pesticides and inhumane conditions that their average life expectancy is reduced to 49 years. We're paying in new cancers, allergies, asthma, reproductive and developmental disorders—the list goes on and on.

Few of us would want to return to hunting and gathering as a means of securing our food. It's not possible today for most of us to grow our own food. But for many who are paying the price of diet-related illness, the cost of all that cheap food has been too high, and the "progress" of our modern food system has gone too far.

As this book powerfully illustrates, the food fight for our species now is the battle to regain much of what we've lost to that progress. Indeed, what we've come to call the Standard American Diet scarcely qualifies as food at all. Rather it's comprised of food-like products that are laced with chemicals, pesticides, hormones, antibiotics, genetically modified organisms, and stunning amounts of added sugar. (The average American now eats more than 150 pounds of added sugar each year, while less than 5% of our population is consuming the recommended amount of fiber.)

The results of this dietary "progress" have been disastrous. More than 2/3 of us are now overweight or obese, and heart disease and stroke are killing more than 700,000 people every year. Our children are affected, too. Where fewer than 2% of America's kids had a chronic health condition in the 1960s, today more than 25% of them do. And one in three American children is expected to get diabetes.

The Great American Food Fight does a brilliant job of revealing how all of these conditions are directly linked to food and to the food choices that are so often made for us, not by us. It exposes hidden dangers in what we're eating and indicts the corporate actions and governmental inaction that have made our diets so lethal. But it's also filled with solutions. Practical suggestions for eating healthier right now as well as simple but powerful ways that each of us can join the fight to return real food choice to consumers. .

There's a lot wrong with our industrial food system, but the hope of fixing it isn't an impossible dream. In fact, the revolution is already building. Our own Food Revolution Network, at work since 2012, now has more than 250,000 members. Many other organizations are also working to transform the food system and the results are starting to show.

Since 1987, organic food sales in the United States have increased over 26-fold, and consumption of feedlot beef has dropped by more than 19 percent. In the last ten years, farmers' markets have increased over three-fold, and sales of natural foods have grown to be a $100 billion industry. Meanwhile, in 2015, McDonalds closed 700 restaurants. Change can come. Together we can make it happen.

I'm proud to welcome Dr. Baldasare and his staff to the revolution and to introduce this book as a tool for achieving our shared goal of sustainable, humane, and conscious food. *The Great American Food Fight* is a clear and and thoughtful look at what's gone wrong and why millions of people are suffering needlessly. And it's a powerful invitation to step into a new food future.

Preface

I never meant to write this book. Well, not such a *big book* anyway. Initially I thought I'd whip out something really concise and manageable—a pamphlet that I could give to those patients who came to me actively seeking information about diet and nutrition. I needed something for those who asked me for advice, but also something for those who didn't. Something also for those patients who were sadly unaware that diet had anything at all to do with their aches, pains, or lack of mobility.

To be truthful there were more and more of these in the last years—patients who were overweight, obese, or morbidly obese. Patients whose treatments were also complicated by diabetes, hypertension, and the coronary conditions that so often accompany obesity. In the last decades health care professionals of every stripe have had to confront this tide of overweight or obese patients and to adapt their practices to it. Specialization in the treatment of obesity through behavioral, cognitive, surgical or pharmaceutical therapies has now become commonplace, but even where obesity isn't the central focus, more and more health care professionals have felt the need to integrate additional services into their wellness programs. My own practice had already expanded to include exercise classes and an annual 90-day Fitness Challenge. Maybe I couldn't do much more, but at least I could commit to writing down some simple strategies for preventing obesity. Strategies, I imagined, that wouldn't involve much more than employing simple common sense.

Almost three years later, I'm amazed at the naiveté with which I began this project. I had no clear notion of how incredibly complicated, or how political, the subject of modern nutrition has become. And almost everything I thought I knew about obesity was wrong.

As many still are, I was originally convinced that the obesity epidemic was rooted in sloth and gluttony. I conceded that stress and other psychological problems sometimes led to overindulgence, and that genetics, for some, was a factor. Generally, though, my private thoughts echoed the public positions taken by today's big food manufacturers: We Americans get fat simply because we make poor individual choices. Because we're too lazy to get enough exercise. Because we succumb to a willful ignorance about good nutrition and we generally fail to take responsibility for our own personal health.

For those who believe this, as I once did, our national character explains a lot about why we lead the world in developing the so-called "diseases of civilization." What it doesn't explain is why the rest of the world gets fat, and sick, too, when we export our diet. And it doesn't even come close to explaining the explosion in allergies, reproductive disorders, gastrointestinal disorders, learning disabilities and many types of cancers.

While that picture of the lazy, slothful American works well for the food manufacturers and their lobbies who would deny their own responsibility in our national obesity scourge, the truth is that far too many of our food choices are made for us, not by us. The struggle to eat healthily has become anything but a simple challenge. In fact, it has become a battle in which many powerful forces are aligned against us. A few of those forces include the difficulty of teasing out sound, factual nutritional information from the contradictory, false, or deliberately misleading propaganda of food conglomerates and their related lobbies and associations. There's the enormous influence of the fast food industry and junk food marketers on all of us, but especially our children—an influence that now extends into the school day itself. There's the fact that American consumers must deal with a chaotic and inconsistent food labeling system which leaves us confused without providing the fundamental information that we have the right to know. Finally, there are the farm and tax policies that subsidize the very foods which make us sick and directly contribute to the obesity epidemic and to rising health care costs.

Where I had originally envisioned a small pamphlet, encouraging readers to make better food "choices" and gently chiding them to exercise more, I ended up with something very different. Rather than adding to the "you're too fat, you're too lazy, you're too ignorant" memes that are neither helpful nor truthful, this has become a book that tries to expose the ways that the American consumer has been victimized, exploited, and maligned in the global obesity epidemic.

My aim has been to explain how many of our food choices are being made without our knowledge and to pull back the curtain on the nutritional misinformation that continues to be disseminated to the public without scientific support. Most importantly I hope to offer specific and immediate help for families in reading between the lines of food labeling, in understanding food dangers, and eating as safely as possible while, together, we bring about change.

While I have some regrets about adding to the proliferation of military metaphors, I cannot see this as anything other than a battle. It's one that must be waged on many fronts and one which we absolutely must win if we and our children are to have long, healthy lives.

Chapter 1. The Battle of Our Lives

It's been a dubious competition—this race to maintain our status as fattest country on earth. In a stunning display of American exceptionalism we've done a pretty good job, for at least the last twenty years anyway, of holding on to that No. 1 spot. The title, however, has recently been lost to Mexico, whose adult obesity rate (32.8 percent) has now edged out our own of 31.8. We're starting to see some competition from other countries as well.

It's hard to call this good news. But reminders of our lack of progress in combatting epidemic obesity have been grim and relentless for decades. It's tempting to seize on almost any development as a hopeful sign of a turning tide. The Centers for Disease Control (CDC) has lent encouragement, too, in suggesting that the overall rise in obesity may be stabilizing. In particular populations, and in sites most dedicated to confronting the problem, obesity rates have declined. Specifically among children ages 2 to 4 in households eligible for food assistance in the Women, Infants and Children (WIC) program.[1]

Given what we know about poverty as a risk factor for obesity, declining rates among the youngest and poorest children may be a genuinely positive sign. But it's much too soon to celebrate.

Where obesity rates may be stabilizing among some groups, the numbers of us most likely to experience the most adverse effects of obesity-related diseases like Type 2 diabetes, heart disease, cancer and other chronic health problems is simply skyrocketing. For vulnerable baby boomers, the obesity rate is above 30 percent in 41 states and about 40 percent in Louisiana and Alabama. For women over 60 the increase has been significant, up 20% since 2003.[2] And the number of Americans with severe obesity—those who are 100 pounds or more over a healthy weight—has soared, increasing by about 70% from 2000 to 2010. [3] The growth of those groups at greatest risk of health complications is increasing at an even greater rate than the rate of obesity.

Children, too, are part of this troubling trend. In 2014, a group of North Carolina researchers found the number of severely obese kids to be rising also. The NC team used the same data that the CDC had used to reach their encouraging conclusions about stabilizing obesity rates among kids, but the NC team extended their own research from 1999 to 2012. Their results, when extending the data out to 14 years, showed no decline. On the contrary they found jumps, among both boys and girls, in rates of obesity and severe obesity. [4]

"We need to be cautious," said lead researcher Asheley Cockrell Skinner, "about reports that say obesity is declining and assume things are better."

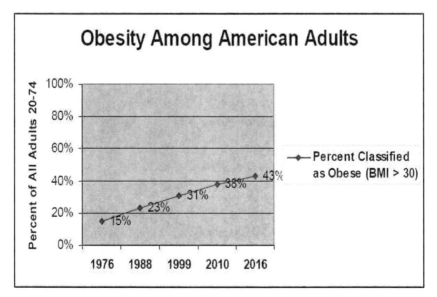

There may be a hollow victory in learning that the rest of the world is starting to put on weight as fast as we Americans, but no real corner has been turned in the battle against obesity. Since 2001, when the Surgeon General first launched the federal initiative to lower the US rate to 15% of the adult population, no state has met the target. Not a single one. And no real success stories have been reported in the past 33 years. The decades-long federal obesity initiative still has a perfect record of failure.

And the bad news doesn't end here. While our title of fattest nation may have been lost, we've begun laying claim to another global distinction. We're rapidly becoming the sickest nation on earth. An examination of historical trends reaching back for decades reveals a strikingly consistent and pervasive pattern of inferior health and earlier death for Americans. As a population we're not getting healthier. On the contrary, we're getting fatter, and sicker, and we're dying younger.

Fatter, Sicker, Dying Younger

While US citizens represent only 5% of the world's population, we consume 50 to 60% of all the world's manufactured drugs and spend more on health care than any other nation on the planet. Yet, despite that flood of drugs and money, Americans come in dead last in comparisons to other affluent nations in terms of health and mortality.[5]

Even some of those advantages that we've come to take for granted as US citizens—like the steady rise in life expectancy during the past two centuries—seems to have come to an end. Especially in the nation's rural counties, and particularly for women. Our position in comparison to other countries with the lowest infant mortality rates appears to be worsening also.

Perhaps the most obvious indicator of our failing national health, however, is in the numbers of us who are falling victim to debilitating, long-term chronic diseases. Almost half of us suffer from at least two of nine chronic conditions: hypertension, heart disease, diabetes, cancer, stroke, chronic bronchitis, emphysema, current asthma and kidney disease. Since the mid-1990s, the number of Americans suffering from at least three of these chronic illnesses has nearly doubled. Even the most cursory examination of how these illnesses affect us as a nation seem cause for despair.

Diabetes

About 29 million of us are now under medical treatment for **Type 2 diabetes**, a four-fold increase since 1980. And that staggering number doesn't even include the millions more who are walking our streets as yet undiagnosed. (The CDC estimates that one in four people with diabetes don't even know it.) An additional 79 million other Americans, suffering from Metabolic Syndrome, are in a pre-diabetic state.

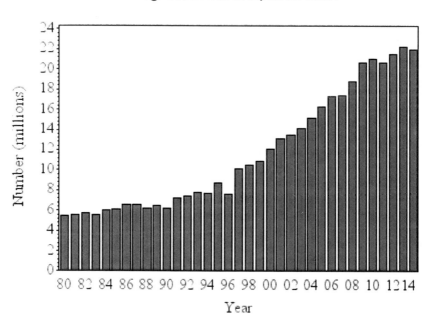

Diagnosed Diabetes, 1980-2014

Predictions for the future are grim, too. Forty percent of Americans born from 2000 to 2011 will develop diabetes, double the risk of those born a decade earlier. As the number of patients increases, so will the burden on the U.S. health-care system.

Cardiovascular Disease

The U.S. death rate from **ischemic heart disease** is the second highest among comparable, high-income peer countries. By age 50 Americans have a less favorable cardiovascular risk profile than our peers in Europe. We're more likely to develop and die from cardiovascular disease than older adults in other high-income countries. According to the American Heart Association (AHA) statistics, there are 53 million Americans with cardiovascular diseases, which includes arteriolosclerosis, high blood pressure, and strokes.

Cancer

While the number of people getting **cancer** in 1900 was about 1 in 33, today it's 1 in 2.5. The U.S. incidence rate for cancer is the fourth highest of the 17 peer countries to which we're most comparable. For some types of cancer, we're much closer to the top. We rank second highest, for example, in rates of breast cancer. And the future doesn't look so good either.

The World Health Organization predicts that new cancer cases will increase 70% over the next two decades as more nations adopt our western diet. Half of those cases, says the WHO, could be prevented by diet. Colon, breast, endometrium, liver, kidney, esophagus, gastric, pancreatic, prostate, gallbladder, and leukemia, are some, but not all, of the cancers that epidemiologists have linked to obesity.

Indeed, cancer and obesity have been called the major epidemics of the century. That's no coincidence. While the biological mechanisms underlying the relationship between cancer and obesity are not well understood, it's clear that these epidemics are not independent. Diet causes cancer.

Other Illnesses

Even though the big three—cancer, CVD, and diabetes—tend to dominate discussions of rising US health care costs, they are not the only indicators of our failing national health. Other illnesses, once rare, are now common, with some approaching epidemic levels.

Chronic digestive disorders like Irritable Bowel Syndrome (IBS), Crohn's disease, diverticulitis, celiac disease and colitis, are on the rise, especially among young patients, aged 18 to 44. Estimates suggest that 20 million of us suffer from these conditions.

A rarity before the mid-1990s, **allergies** are now the fifth most common chronic disease. Both skin and food allergies have been steadily increasing for more than a decade, with sufferers being preponderantly children under the age of 18.

Children, too, are increasingly the victims of **asthma**, almost unheard of a few generations ago, but now the most common chronic childhood disease. Asthma incidence is not only increasing, especially among children under age 6, but the disease is becoming more severe.

Our children, indeed, may be the greatest victims of our industrialized food system. Mental illnesses that once hovered in the shadows of our collective awareness now loom large. Neurological conditions and developmental disorders, like **autism**, are increasing in such epidemic proportions that terms like "plague" don't seem at all inappropriate.

Many of these diseases and conditions, at least in the public consciousness, don't seem directly related to diet. Yet, as this book will show, they are. Diseases as seemingly unrelated to food as asthma and **Alzheimer's** are directly linked to the Standard American Diet (SAD) and the obesity pandemic it has created. Studies have shown that being overweight or obese increases sensitivity to indoor air pollution in urban children with asthma. An emerging body of research links Alzheimer's disease to insulin resistance, in turn linked to excess sweetener consumption. [6] In other discussions in these pages we'll see, again and again, the science that is connecting specific illness to specific ingredients or specific practices in modern food production.

It's hard to deny that our food is killing us. But why is this happening? Is it simply because we're eating too much of it?

Choosing to Be Fat and Sick?

The national debate over what is driving the public health crisis of obesity has raged for decades. Social surveys, however, consistently suggest that most citizens understand obesity to be a matter of "individual responsibility." This is certainly the attitude embraced by food manufacturers themselves. The thinking goes that those who succumb to the preventable suffering of obesity—and the many other diseases that follow in its wake—do so as a result of their own poor "lifestyle" choices. They are somehow *choosing* to be fat and sick.

Choices, however, don't occur in a vacuum. There are some serious problems with conceiving of the obesity epidemic as a mass failure of personal responsibility.

The notion that obesity is about personal choice rests on at least three fundamental assumptions:

1) That the ability to eat healthily is available to all of us.

2) That we have sound and accurate information on which to base our food choices.

3) That our choices are not being influenced by undue pressure from corporate, government or other sources.

None of these assumptions are true. They're not even close to the truth. The truth is that our current food system exerts enormous and insidious influence on our choices. It works stealthily to steer us into choices we don't know we're making. It operates to conceal what we're buying, and eating, to promote the unhealthiest foods to us and our children, to subsidize those foods through our tax system, and even to chemically engineer them for physiological addiction.

In what amounts to an eye blink of human history, a small handful of corporations, with the cooperation and consent of government, has so reshaped our national food system that the consumers of an entire nation are now digging their graves with their forks.

That very same food system is being exported to the rest of the world at such a lightning speed, and with so little political resistance, that our national epidemic will soon become global pandemic. In the context of our current food system, premature deaths, chronic disease and endlessly escalating health care costs are really not preventable. They're inevitable.

> In the context of our current food system, premature deaths, chronic disease and endlessly escalating health care costs are really not preventable. They're inevitable.

Except for those who are affluent and resourceful enough to manage to eat outside the system, there's no such thing as free choice when it comes to food. Most American consumers don't have the luxury of eating outside the system. Within it, we have far less control than we realize.

Narrowing Food Choice

The aisles of a large, modern supermarket may contain upwards of 40,000 products. That's a number that sounds not just ample, but almost daunting in the shopping decisions it represents. With so much to choose from, one might think, today's consumer has virtually unlimited opportunities to make informed choices for good health and good value.

Those choices, however, are not nearly so abundant and varied as they seem. Our grocery stores may be getting larger and larger, but real consumer choices are actually being narrowed.

Where our grandparents often bought groceries at a local level, from neighborhood stores or from state, sometimes regional supermarket chains, today's consumers are buying groceries from national and international mega-retailers, from big box stores and supercenters. Intense consolidation throughout the grocery industry has limited not just where we can shop, but what we can buy. In 2012, for example, more than half of all our food dollars went to one of only four retailers.

For all the different brands and food names on the market, only a handful of companies dominate the industry. Where grocery shelves seem packed with a bewildering array of food products, those products actually come from a very limited number of foods, re-configured, re-packaged, and re-branded to present an illusion of choice. These are the highly processed, salt and sugar-loaded convenience products found in the center of the store. They are the same products—made from a very few plant and animal sources—that produce the most profit for food manufacturers while being the least healthy for consumers.

And yet even that center-of-the-store bounty is a mirage. Where consumers often believe they are choosing among competitors, they are often only selecting from products made by the same company. Often made in the same factory. In every link of the food chain, from farm to fork, consolidation of our food supply has reduced us to false choices, blind choices, or no choice at all.

> In every link of the food chain, from farm to fork, consolidation of our food supply has reduced us to false choices, blind choices, or no choice at all.

Any number of exercises can reveal the limitations in personal choice that our industrial food system has imposed. Try, for example, to buy a food not grown from corporate seeds. Try to find bread not manufactured from a government-subsidized grain. Try to buy a cereal that doesn't list sugar and salt as a main ingredient, or one not manufactured by the big Four—Kellogg, General Mills, PepsiCo, or Post, which represent 79.9% of all brands. Choose a beef product that didn't come from one of the four producers who control 80% of the market.

None of these exercises, however, will really expose the place where American consumers have been most seriously deprived of choice. For a real challenge, try to buy any of the tens of thousands of food plant varieties grown in this country during the last century that have now become extinct as a result of industrial monoculture.

Among the long list of choices that are no longer available to us is the nearly 93 percent of lost lettuce varieties, over 96 percent of sweet corn, more than 95 percent of tomato, and almost 98 percent of asparagus varieties. And those are but a few examples.

The U.N. Food and Agriculture Organization (FAO) estimates that more than three-quarters of agricultural genetic diversity was lost in this past century. Astonishingly, a full 95 percent of the calories we eat today now come from only 30 varieties of plants.

This shocking loss of native diversity represents not only an environmental disaster but also a staggering reduction in food choices available to us and to future generations. And that is only the beginning of the ways that Big Food, Big Agriculture, and Big Government are manipulating food choices.

The sad truth is that for every repackaged, re-branded, and heavily marketed product that appears on supermarket shelves, consumers have lost the opportunity to choose from a hundred—perhaps a thousand—varieties of plants that our grandparents once enjoyed.

Subsidizing Death and Disease

Few American families can ignore price when buying food. For many it's the primary consideration. We've got lots of help, though, when it comes to influencing our decisions about where we put those limited food dollars. That help comes from the administration of national farm policies that keep junk food cheap, effectively using our own tax dollars to subsidize death and disease.

Uncle Sam wants you, and your children, to eat a diet that is excessively high in grains, sugars, and factory-farmed meats. That's why he pays billions of taxpayer dollars to a very few, very large corporate farmers to grow an extremely short list of agricultural commodities.

We can't, of course, actually eat all of these commodities. Only about 1% of the national corn crop, for example, is the sweet corn we directly consume. Most of these crops are processed into additives like corn syrup, high fructose corn syrup, corn starch, and soy oils (which are frequently processed further into hydrogenated vegetable oils). By no mere coincidence are these additives the key ingredients of the food that is making us fat, and sick.

The perversity of this arrangement has been made abundantly clear in the reports issued by the U.S. Public Interest Research Group (U.S. PIRG.) Their report, titled "Apples to Twinkies," notes that produce like oranges or spinach receives no regular federal funding, with the single exception of apples, on which the government spent about one hundredth of one percent (0.001) of its agricultural subsidy money between 1995 and 2010. The four common junk food additives, however, were subsidized to the tune of $18.2 billion. [7]

The newest U.S. PIRG report puts those numbers into perspective by noting that the money spent on junk food subsidies since 1995 is enough to buy nearly 52 *billion* Twinkies. Enough Twinkies to encircle the globe 132 times. (The recently re-engineered Twinkie, by the way, is made with 17 taxpayer-subsidized ingredients, including corn starch, corn syrup and vegetable shortening.) By contrast, the money for the only fruit or vegetable that gets any significant subsidies would buy each taxpayer less than half an apple.

The illustrations here provide another way to look at this disparity and its influence on national health. The first graphic shows the new dietary guidance symbol, MyPlate, created by the U.S. Department of Agriculture (USDA). It was designed to suggest a healthy proportional ratio of food group choices to be consumed in a meal.

As you can see, MyPlate encourages us to make vegetables and grains almost equally important. It recommends that fruits provide almost a quarter of a healthy meal.

The second graphic, however, shows the message that our government is really sending in terms of the food groups it actually subsidizes. Those subsidies create the completely artificial price inequalities that enable highly processed junk food to undersell much more nutritious, but unsubsidized, fruits and vegetables. Those subsidies are also the reason that recession-battered consumers "choose" the lower-priced junk food.

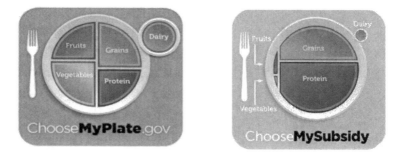

American consumers are caught in the classic vicious cycle. We are spending taxpayer dollars to make junk food cheaper, which makes us fatter and sicker, thereby driving up healthcare costs, which drive up our taxes even further.

Promoting Death and Disease

Few parents would knowingly stand still while a deluge of advertising promoted opiates, narcotics, or other addictive substances to their children. Yet we're allowing the processed food industry to do something quite like that in targeting our children with over 40,000 advertisements each year, of which 72% are for candy, cereal, and fast foods.

The collective pester power of the fast food industry alone comes purchased with annual advertising budgets exceeding $4.2 billion. (That's billion!). McDonald's U.S. spend alone is estimated at more than $1 billion dollars per year. And these figures don't even include the marketing of individually branded items that may be part of a fast food meal. Coca-Cola, for example, spends another 2 billion each year.

Highly integrated marketing campaigns, honed over thirty years, create lifelong brand loyalties in our children. They're created through the distribution of toys as premiums for children's meals, colorful onsite playgrounds, birthday party packages, the appearances of licensed characters and other child-friendly allures, and they're reinforced by an absolute tsunami of TV, radio, print, and internet advertising. Online websites, designed to look like entertainment for children, develop mega data on children consumers.

It's a marketing strategy that works extraordinarily well to make loyal brand advocates of the very youngest customers. How well does it work? In research conducted at Stanford University, pre-schoolers rated food in the familiar McDonald's packaging up to six times more appetizing than the identical snacks packaged in plain wrappers.

The brand affinity was not reserved just for fast foods, either. The children even found that milk and carrots tasted better when they believed these were made by a big brand.[8]

The extent to which a child's taste preferences can be influenced by advertising may be dismaying, but it's not likely to shock most parents. In a survey commissioned by the Rudd Center for Food Policy and Obesity at Yale University, 40 percent of parents reported that their children asked to go to McDonald's at least once a week, and 15 percent of parents of two to five-year-olds said that their children harangue them for a Mickey D's trip *every single day*.[9]

Racial and Ethnic Targeting

While all children are fair game in the branding and bonding efforts of food marketing, some children are of particular interest, especially to the big fast food companies. There's a disturbing racial component in the disproportionate targeting by fast food restaurants of ethnic and minority youth.

Fast food ads, for example, appear more frequently during African American-targeted TV programming than during general audience programming. On Spanish-language television networks, fast food advertisements comprise nearly half of all ads. Billboards for fast food restaurants appear significantly more often in low-income African

American and Latino neighborhoods. Fast food restaurants located in poorer African American neighborhoods also promote less-healthful foods and have more in-store advertisements compared to restaurants in more affluent, predominantly white neighborhoods. This racial and ethnic targeting adds another economic element, as well as a moral component, to the vicious cycle in which many consumers are already caught. Obesity-related hypertension occurs at much higher rates among African-Americans, and obesity-related diabetes occurs at higher rates among Mexican Americans.

For the past thirty years the food industry has aggressively marketed to children while vigorously resisting federal efforts to change its products and practices. Commercial interests consistently override the health concerns of our children.

Schools for Sale

While it's nearly impossible to distract our children from this pester power when we're around them, fast food and junk food marketing even extends into the school day itself. More and more schools, in exchange for desperately needed funds, are contracting with major soft drink and fast food companies to advertise and sell their products to children in the school. Over a third of elementary schools, half of middle schools and almost three-quarters of high schools currently have contracts that give companies monopoly rights to sell soft drinks in their buildings in exchange for a percentage of the revenues.

In return for loans of satellite dishes, VCRs, and TV equipment, children in many schools are obliged to watch shows accompanied by commercials, primarily for junk food and video games, during the school day. The commercials are compulsory in this arrangement, as teachers have no ability to turn them off. The best known example of this is Channel One News, an "educational" TV program shown in schools that includes two minutes of advertising. Channel One is shown in over 12,000 middle and high schools across the United States, reaching 8 million students.[10]

Advertising on school grounds is also common, with beverage and snack food advertisements plastering book covers and other educational materials, as well as school sports field fences, gymnasiums and stadiums. At least seven states have overturned long-standing laws that prohibit advertising on school buses. And the latest in ad creep? School bus radio.

Unfortunately, our school lunch programs are not much of counterweight to this onslaught by way of either influence or example. Menus in most school lunch programs are too high in salt and sugar and too low in fiber and nutrient-rich fruits, vegetables, whole grains, and legumes. Despite efforts to serve healthier meals to school children, roughly half of U.S. elementary school kids can still buy junk food at school. Around a fifth of high schools also offer brand-name fast foods like Pizza Hut or Taco Bell. Multiple studies have also found that fast food chains are clustered disproportionately around schools where they can cater to students at the beginning and end of the school day and to the 5 to 15 percent of high school students who leave the campus for lunch.

When you add all this school day propaganda to traditional afterschool TV advertising, to cross-promotions and product placement in movies and video games, and now to the digital, and increasingly social, marketing delivered on the internet and through mobile technologies, we parents are left with almost no spin-free zone where we can even attempt to inoculate our children against fast food and junk food hype.

Disguising Death and Disease

The starting point for making good decisions must always be good information. Yet, as more and more of us are coming to realize, much of the information that we need to make the healthiest, and safest, food choices is obscured or deliberately kept from us by those who profit from our lack of awareness. The struggle to label genetically modified food is the most egregious, but it's only one example. Despite the fact that food products have never displayed so many symbols and statements claiming nutrition and health benefits, consumers are justifiably confused by much of that information. In the regulatory chaos that governs food labeling, manufacturers are happy to exploit that confusion.

The importance to public health of clear, truthful, scientifically valid food labeling was acknowledged in 1990 with implementation of the Nutrition Labeling and Education Act. A quarter of a century later, an entire industry has emerged intent on disguising and obscuring food ingredients and confusing and defrauding the consumer.

The struggle to simply know what we're eating is a battle that the American food consumer, for decades, has been consistently losing. As the discussions in this book—on additives, packaging and health claims—will show, food labeling has become an exercise in deception. Much food production, especially animal agriculture, is almost entirely opaque to the consumer. Nutrition science is too often co-opted by corporate bankrolled academics whose "research" invariably benefits the products and practices of Big Food.[11] Our own government is complicit in allowing food industry lobbyists to manipulate and control the discourse on food policy.

Transparency is the enemy of Big Food. To the corporate food industry, answers to questions about what's in our food, where it comes from, how it's produced, and its effect on our bodies, are simply none of our business.

The burden of personal responsibility in making food choices becomes considerably heavier when an entire industry is bent on disguising and confusing, obscuring and defrauding. We can't choose wisely when we don't even know what we're choosing.

Engineering Death and Disease

The discovery that cigarette makers were intentionally manipulating nicotine content to make their products more addictive enraged the general public and led to major legislative reforms in regard to tobacco sales and advertising. But the food industry has long been guilty of the same tactics.

The hyper palatable foods that are passed to us through a fast-food drive in window, and the highly processed food-like products that fill the center aisles of the grocery, are nothing if not triumphs of modern chemistry. Their appearance, aromas, flavors, and textures are laboratory-designed to manipulate our neurological responses. They are engineered to excite the brain's reward centers while overriding our bodies' hunger/satiety signals, frustrating our ability to feel satisfied. Excessive calorie intake is promoted simply by the fact that that the original whole food from which many processed foods are made is so broken down that it lacks sufficient nutrition to signal fullness to our brains.

We've been slow to admit that food addiction is real. But there's enough evidence now to demonstrate that the same biological mechanics that drive people into drug addiction are behind the compulsion to overeat. Indeed, we now have more scientific verification for physical craving as a dynamic of food addiction than existed with regard to alcoholism and other drug addictions when they were first designated as substance use disorders.

Personal responsibility has a role in everyone's diet. But it's time to acknowledge that many foods today are laboratory-designed to encourage us to eat more than we really want.

In many discussions in this book, but particularly those in Chapter 10 on Sugar and Artificial Sweeteners, we'll see obesity in the larger context of our highly obesogenic food environment. For a great many of us, overeating is a biological challenge. It's one made much more difficult by national policies that encourage unhealthy eating, by the food industry's aggressive marketing tactics, and by sophisticated chemical engineering that essentially turns food into drugs.

Fighting Back

As fewer and fewer big players have come to dominate our industrialized food system, real food choice for the consumer is disappearing. We don't really know what we're eating anymore. In the absence of sufficient testing or monitoring to determine human health impact, we don't even know that it's safe. While the corporate food sector gets better at protecting its bottom line, the interests of the food-buying public are being ignored. Our environment is being degraded. Animals are being cruelly abused. Our tax dollars are being squandered. As a nation we're getting fatter, sicker, and dying younger.

I, for one, believe that these trends must be reversed. And I know I'm not alone. Today's consumers are slowly waking up to the fact that our food supply and reality-based conversation about it has been hijacked. We've become suspicious of nutrition messaging from the food industry. We're losing confidence in government to safeguard consumers' interest over corporate ones. And we're getting really weary of food manufacturers and their lobbyists controlling the debate and framing the issues surrounding the obesity epidemic in ways that relieve them of all responsibility.

As much as we Americans enjoy the convenience of our corporatized, industrialized food system, we're no longer willing to be held hostage to it. We're getting smarter about how our food choices have been controlled. We're starting to take back the conversation about the obesity epidemic and to push back on the guilt trippers who suggest that our laziness, our ignorance, and our apathy—even our national character—is responsible for the national health crisis we're experiencing.

I'm convinced that concern on many food issues is about to achieve critical mass. The GMO labeling initiatives, Prop. 37 in California, and Prop 52 in Washington, were not successful in getting genetically modified foods labeled in those states. Those defeats, however, produced some surprising victories. They have galvanized consumers and created new food activists not just in the US, but all over the globe. Here in the US statewide labelling initiatives are still going strong. To date, over 70 bills have been introduced in over 30 states to require GE labeling or prohibition of genetically engineered foods. Food companies are choosing to opt-out of GMO ingredients in the manufacturing of their food products due to consumer demand.

Retailers are doing the same.

This book was written in the fervent hope of moving us closer to the critical mass—that place where change will come. Its primary goal is to separate the objective science from the corporate spin and to shine some light on the food battles that we absolutely must win.

Yet, while accurate information is certainly the starting point for empowering individuals and families to make better food choices, it's only a beginning. To bring about the comprehensive, long-term changes that will give us and our children a better chance at a long and healthy life, we will need to fight on many fronts. Some of those fronts are legislative, while others are market-based. But elected officials will never be able to withstand the influence of big business and their lobbyists without the American consumer at their backs. And there is no incentive for food manufacturers to change unless the consumer demands change.

Toward that end we've also included information on many volunteer, non-profit and consumer advocacy groups who are working to educate us on particular food and nutrition issues and to effect policy changes that will make our food product systems safer, healthier, and more transparent. The hope is that each reader will find at least one battlefront on which they are willing to stand and fight.

It would not be wise to underestimate the forces that we're up against in the Great American Food Fight. But I don't think there's cause for despair. As we get smarter, we can bring about immediate changes in our individual households and begin to teach and model healthier eating for our children. If we get together, we can bring about positive changes in public policy. Many groups opposed to today's food system are already pursuing litigation, pressuring branded food companies, and initiating legislation to change how the system operates. Local, national, and global grassroots movements are already pointing us toward solutions for sustainable food and agricultural policies. Change can come. But we're going to have to fight for it.

Eating in the Meantime

In the meantime we have to eat. Every day we have to make food choices for ourselves and our families. Let's start where we all start—in the supermarket, the local grocery, the farmers markets and co-ops, where we buy apples, steaks, and baby formula. Our food fight starts there, in better understanding what we're buying and eating.

At the conclusion of each chapter in this book, you'll find an *Eating in the Meantime* section like this one distilling the preceding chapter into the actionable advice and steps you can take, right now, to begin making better, safer, choices for yourself and your family.

At the end of the book you'll also find:

- **Notes** to the scholarly studies, reports and popular articles cited in this volume.

- A list of **Additional Resources**, giving you suggestions for expanding your knowledge through web, print, and video resources that provide more in-depth information on particular subjects. This resource list also includes the names and web addresses of many governmental, consumer watchdog, food activists, and non-profit organizations that are working to educate consumers, investigate family health threats, or disseminate information on specific food and nutrition issues.

  Every attempt has been made to eliminate commercially branded sites and those marketing entities that sell products or earn a commission from products they review.

- An **Appendix**, which contains many handy charts and tables for quick reference

- An **Index,** through which you can quickly re-discover references or discussions on a specific topic

Printable versions of much of this material, more articles and news on food fight battlefronts, and links for fighting back can be found on our website at www.GreatAmericanFoodFight.com.

Chapter 2. All the Pretty Packages: Buyer Beware

That old maxim that goes "you can't judge a book by its cover" can apply, by analogy, to food. Especially to the processed and manufactured foods that make up almost 80% of American diets. In many cases what's inside that box, can, or package that we purchase at the supermarket is completely concealed from us. We're left to rely on the pretty package, its pictures and words, to know what's really inside.

It's the words, of course, those descriptors of the package's contents, its ingredients and their nutritional values, which should carry the most weight in influencing our food shopping decisions. Yet, as every parent who's ever shopped with a toddler knows, you don't have to be able to read to have an opinion in the grocery store. Kids know what they like, and they know because the package tells them.

We grown-ups, of course, know better. As literate adults, we're not nearly so susceptible to the allure of pretty packaging. We don't judge our food by its cover. Or do we?

Getting Past the Package

The American supermarket is a stimulating—sometimes an over-stimulating, place. In a typical grocery store there may be as many as 45,000 items all clamoring for our attention and competing for our grocery dollar. It's only natural that we're attracted to the bright combinations of colors, the interesting logos, the clever topography and art. It's natural, too, to forget that everything we see there has been through a design process, subjected to focus groups and professional copywriters—a marketing process that we will pay for at the cash register, in many instances at a value many times greater than that of the food or beverage inside.

Take, for example, the new chocolate milk bottle introduced by Nestlé in 2000. Nestlé was taking its NesQuik product from a traditional tabletop carton to a completely new extended shelf life package that would not only require the company to purchase new filling and handling equipment, but would demand that the product be merchandised and distributed differently. Even with the support of its own internal research efforts, the new package would be a calculated gamble. It was one, however, that paid off spectacularly.

The new packaging virtually made NesQuik a new product. Sales increased approximately 220% in its first year on the market. Dean Lindsay, the designer of the package, quotes then-president Edward Meara of the Nestlé Beverage Division, as directly crediting the sales spike to the new "16-ounce contoured, easy-grip, car-holder convenient plastic bottle, dressed head-to-toe in a full body shrink-sleeve label."[12]

I don't mean to disparage Nestlé's success or its bold marketing move. I'm not even suggesting that consumers who bought their chocolate milk in contoured, easy-grip, car-holder- convenient, shrink-wrapped bottles were being taken in. And while issues of over-packaging have environmental implications for all us, that's still not the main focus here. I've related the Nestlé example because it's a good illustration of what food manufacturers know all too well. Quite often, the package *is* the product. We buy the cover, not the book.

Certainly an important first step in getting better value for our food dollars, both nutritionally and economically, is learning to get past the package. As citizens, consumers, and parents we need to develop not just a healthy skepticism, but a tough, informed cynicism about food marketing and packaging. Those pretty packages are interesting and alluring, but they are not designed with our health, or our budgets, in mind. Sometimes our kids will want to influence our purchasing decisions. And sometimes we'll let them. There will sometimes be instances when the demands of convenience, portability, or storage may justify buying the cover not the book. But we should do it with our eyes wide open.

I'm often dismayed, even in my own family, and even with myself, at how mindlessly we succumb to expensive and unnecessary packaging. Must our chocolate milk *really* be car-holder convenient? Will bite-sized, foil-encased, cheese cubes really save me *that* much time? Do we really *need* individually wrapped baking potatoes?

Packaging Sneaks and Cheats

While the size of packaging may not seem immediately relevant in a book focusing on nutrition and health, I'm of the opinion that it's plenty important. When you're paying for air, your food dollar is being wasted.

There are few of us who have not encountered the irritation, and disappointment, of discovering that a bag, jar, or box contained much less than we were expecting. Sometimes we're not really being shortchanged. There are functional reasons for "slack fill" in packages, like protecting delicate and breakable contents during transport. But cutting quantity to avoid raising prices is a time-honored tactic for manufacturers in tight economies. And in this one, too, many shoppers are noticing a trend toward stealthily shrinking package sizes. Deloitte's Consumer Food and Product Insight Survey found that nearly almost three-quarters of respondents (74 percent) say the size of some packaged goods is smaller.[13]

Packaging to Price

The practice of manipulating package design or size to disguise price increases is called "packaging to price" and manufacturers are getting very clever at it. Here are just a few techniques that they hope busy shoppers won't notice:

- Changing the shape of the package.

- Reducing the depth, but not the width, of familiar boxes. From the aisle, everything looks the same.

- Distracting from smaller sizes with banners like "New E-Z pour bottle," or "Same Great Taste."

- Describing new, but smaller, packaging as "greener," "future friendly," or with similar terms to suggest that it uses fewer resources in its manufacture.

- Packaging in larger containers, bags, or boxes to conceal product price hikes. The packages may say, "Now, 40% more!" But you're paying 50% more.

- Adding more brine, syrup, or water to foods.

- Packaging in new, visually similar containers, but slightly reducing the content food. Here the "pound" of bacon suddenly weighs 15 ounces and the "pint" of ice cream now contains only 14 ounces.

Black Hole Tactics

While packaging to price can be defended as the simple exercise of free market principles, some "black hole" tactics are especially deceitful. These include

- Adding dimples to the bottom of jars or molded packages

- Including useless partitioning inside packages, or bags inside packages

- Concealing pure emptiness, not evident at purchase, under bubble or blister packaging

Fight Back!

While shopping with a sharp eye and a pocket calculator may be our best defense against shrinking value, we can fight back against black hole tactics in packaging. Send your nominee to *Consumer Reports.org* for its **Black Hole Award**.

You can also file a complaint with the FDA. A list of district complaint coordinators for each state can be found on the FDA website at **www.fda.gov/safety/reportaproblem/consumercomplaintcoor dinators/default.htm.**

Our main protection against deceptive packaging practices like these is in the Fair Packaging and Labeling Act (the FPLA) enacted in 1966. The FPLA legislation, six years in the making, had its roots in consumer anger about many of the deceptive packaging practices that still exist today—slack fill, packaging to price, and the wild proliferation of odd weights and package sizes. The FPLA ultimately did strengthen consumer bargaining power a little. Packages now must provide the name and address of the manufacturer. The statement of net quantity must be conspicuous and readable. Processed foods now must provide a statement of serving size. But the law has been minimally successful at protecting us from those deceptive packaging practices and marketing ploys used by manufacturers to give us as little value for our dollar as possible. FPLA's enforcement of The Fair Packaging and Labeling Act has been largely been ceded to the FDA, which has no power to regulate product downsizing, and the agency's track record on slack fill has been nothing to brag about. [14] It hasn't acted on a slack fill case in six years.

Packaging tricks are serious concerns because they make it so much more difficult for shoppers to make rational decisions with their food dollars. This is certainly one of the fronts in the Great American Food Fight and it's one where, for now, the consumer has few allies in Washington. But the real battle surrounding all those pretty packages is something much more fundamental. It's the struggle to understand what's actually inside them.

> The Principle of *caveat emptor*—"Let the buyer beware"— should not apply to food. We have a right to know what we're eating.

Packaging that cheats us of contents is one thing. Packaging that misleads, or lies outright about what's inside is something else entirely. Accurate labeling is necessary to avoid food intolerances and to prevent life-threatening allergic reactions. It's critical for controlling medical conditions like diabetes and hypertension that are regulated by diet. It's necessary for allowing us to conform to personal ethical convictions and religious practices. Truthful labeling is also important for managing our weight and ensuring that our families' nutritional needs are met. The principle of *caveat emptor*—"Let the buyer beware"—should not apply to food. We have a right to know what we're buying.

Front-of-Pack Labeling

The most informative element on the outside of processed food is the Nutrition Facts Panel, usually found on the back or side of packages. But it's the *front* packaging label, also called the principal display panel, or PDP, that is most likely to be seen by the consumer at the time of purchase. What we see and read on the PDP greatly influences our buying decisions, but even with something as basic as the very name of the product, we're sometimes fooled.

Product Identification

A rose, thought Shakespeare, would smell just as sweet by any other name. I'm not prepared to argue with him. I would argue, however, that what our food is named can influence its smell, its taste, and our perception of its nutritional benefits. A study described in *The Journal of Consumer Research* illustrates the psychological power of simple word choice.

In this study, two groups of participants were presented with the same mixture of vegetables, pasta, salami, and cheese, served on a bed of fresh romaine lettuce. The item was identified as either "salad" or "pasta." When it was called pasta, dieters perceived it as less healthy. In another study, participants were given either a product labeled "fruit chews" or one labeled "candy chews." In results described by the authors, "Dieters perceived the item with an unhealthy name (candy chews) to be less healthful and less tasty than non-dieters. As a result, dieters consumed more of the confections when they were called "fruit chews."[15]

Statement of Identity

The FDA calls the common or usual name of a packaged food, the *statement of identity*. Thus, in the labeling of Campbell's Cream of Chicken with Herbs Soup, the statement of identity is "soup." That seems straightforward enough. Problems arise, however, when so many of the identifiers naming products today are not recognizable as food. The "Twinkie," apparently, was just the beginning of a rush of food-naming inventiveness that shows no signs of slowing down.

Products today can be named simply for their shape (rounds, squares, rolls, bars, twists, stars, curls), for their size (snacks, bites, thins, treats, minis, nibbles), or for their textures, or the sounds we presumably make when we eat them (crisps, crunches, smacks, chewies). My personal favorite is Betty Crocker's line of fruit "Gushers"—a food name that rivals the Twinkie for sheer originality.

These invented or fanciful food names are problematic in several ways. First, because many FDA regulations are written *in reference to* common or usual foods. In a class by itself, a Gusher can't be considered an imitation of another food or deemed nutritionally inferior to one. Secondly, because this food-naming cleverness makes the busy shopper more dependent than ever on information usually found on the back, not the front, of packaging.

> As enlightened consumers, we can learn to look with suspicion on packages promoting products that are hard to identify as food.

There's little hope that food labeling regulations can stay ahead of capitalistic creativity. But there is hope. As enlightened consumers we can learn to look with suspicion on packages promoting products that are hard to identify as food.

Before we toss that beautiful package of Strawberry Splash Fruit Gushers into our cart, we'd do well to turn the package over. Only there will we learn than Strawberry Gushers contain more than 20 ingredients, including Trans fats, 13 grams of sugar, three different food coloring additives, three forms of corn, partially hydrolyzed cottonseed oil, multiple chemical preservatives, some grape juice and pears from concentrate, but alas, no strawberries.

Health Claims

Often what catches our eye on the fronts of processed foods is the manufacturer's promise, or implied promise, of the product's benefit to our family's health. It's very difficult for a parent to ignore statements like "Boost your child's brainpower" or "Support a healthy immune system." While claims like these demonstrably promote sales, research shows that they are poorly understood by the consumer, who often gets an inflated idea of the food's nutritional value. [16]

Some claims on front of pack labeling are indeed evidence-based statements reflecting significant scientific agreement (SSA). Others are just fancy word-smithing bearing little relationship to the products on which they're plastered. It can be very difficult to tell the difference.

Qualified and Unqualified Health Claims

All health claims characterize the relationship of a nutrient to a disease or health-related condition. *Example:* "Eating high fiber grain products may help prevent some cancers." The FDA distinguishes between types of health claims, calling them "qualified" or "unqualified." There's a difference. But it's one often missed by consumers who have actually lost ground in recent years in knowing where the science stands on nutritional issues.

Prior to 2002, the FDA held manufacturers to the strict SSA standard of scientific evidence before approving health claims on food labels. (Again, that's Significant Scientific Agreement.) These would be those claims which most of the scientific community currently supports.

In 1999, however, dietary supplement marketers sued the FDA, arguing that they should be allowed to inform consumers of potential health benefits and that applying only the standards of rigorous scientific evidence interfered with rights of free speech. The court sided with the plaintiffs and thus, rather counter-intuitively, "qualified" health claims (QHCs) became those which must accompanied by a disclaimer or otherwise "qualified."

The FDA now calls those claims that are actually backed by scientific support, "unqualified" because they can stand alone without further explanation or qualification.

Example: "Soluble fiber (whole oats, psyllium seed husk) reduces coronary heart disease risk."

Many nutrition experts believe that qualified health claims have turned the FDA into a pawn of the food industry, allowing ridiculous claims to confuse consumers into buying the wrong kinds of food. While qualified health claims do mean that emerging evidence exists between a food and reduced risk of a disease, the science is not conclusive. The claim, or suggestion of that relationship, is often made on the front of the package, while qualifying disclaimers usually appear in very small print and usually at the bottom of the package.

Structure/Function Claims

Structure/function claims refer to a food's effect on a structure or function in the human body, but not to a disease. *Example:* "Calcium builds strong bones." Manufacturers like to make use of these claims because they don't require the "fine print" notices demanded of qualified health claims, which can turn consumers off.

Structure/function claims are not pre-reviewed or authorized by the FDA. Like qualified health claims, however, they often rely on weak or limited scientific evidence. While the FDA may *ask* food manufacturing companies to submit evidence of scientific substantiation, it has no legal authority to force any company to provide it.

Consumer Confusion over Health Claims

In January 2011 The U.S. Government Accountability Office (GAO) presented to Congress the results of a study analyzing the FDA's oversight of health claims. Unsurprisingly, the GAO found that consumers don't really understand the differences in scientific support between unqualified health claims and qualified health claims.[17] Consumer advocacy groups like the Center for Science in the Public Interest have long been voicing this same complaint, as have many nutrition scientists. Marion Nestle, professor of Nutrition, Food Studies, and Public Health at New York University, and the author of *Food Politics, Safe Food, What to Eat,* and other nutrition books, thinks that we might be better served without any health claims at all. Says Nestle:

> If health claims are allowed on food packages, they should be regulated more strictly according to rigorous, evidence based national standards. Because such standards are inevitably arbitrary and subject to manipulation, consideration should be given to an outright ban on all front-of package claims. Doing so would aid educational efforts to encourage the public to eat whole or minimally processed foods and to read the ingredient lists on processed foods.[18]

Product Endorsements

In a celebrity-obsessed culture, it's not surprising that a picture or signature endorsement of a movie star, model, athlete, or rap star should help to sell food. Since 1934, when Lou Gehrig first appeared on a box of Wheaties, generations of Americans have been eating what their heroes eat. Or at least what we *think* they eat. There's a lot of "pester power" for parents in these celebrity endorsements, even if we're savvy enough to know that the face of Heidi Klum on chewy candies or Sylvester Stallone on instant pudding doesn't say much about nutrition. Where we're much more likely to be taken, however, is with another type of endorsement. This is the endorsement or certification of foods by reputable organizations known to promote research and education in the prevention of disease.

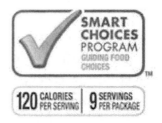

Most consumers are accustomed to seeing the symbols, logos, or slogans of organizations like the American Cancer Society, Diabetes Association, or the American Heart Association on packaging. The Heart Association's "HeartChecked" logo is perhaps the best-known example. These endorsements inspire confidence in buyers who are not aware that such certifications are bought and paid for by food manufacturers.

Marion Nestle has written extensively about how corporate control of the nation's food system limits our choices and threatens our health. In *Food Politics*, she describes the history of how the endorsement practice began as a fund-raising endeavor by the American Heart Association in 1988. (The AHA's HeartChecked logo now goes for $7,500 per product with a $4,500 fee for annual renewals.) The program, says Nestle, "cannot help but raise questions about credibility" and sometimes results in advertisements that are "nutritionally absurd."[19]

A third type of endorsement occurs when companies create their own nutrition criteria and then apply that standard to their own products. You may have seen the logos, seals or stickers for nutrition programs like "Smart Spot," managed by PepsiCo, "Sensible Solutions," owned by Kraft, and the "Smart Choices" system designed by and paid for by many of the nation's top food manufacturers, including Kellogg's, Kraft Foods, ConAgra Foods, Unilever, General Mills, PepsiCo and Tyson Foods.

These self-endorsement labeling systems may encourage families to buy, but some of the choices they certify are highly questionable and have come under criticism from nutritionists. Researchers at Yale University, examining 100 packaged products with the Smart Choices designation, found that more than 60 % of the foods that had received the label did not meet standard nutritional criteria for a healthy food choice.[20] Nestle herself was recently astounded when the green check mark for Smart Choices appeared on Froot Loops cereal.

The Bottom Line: These industry-backed labeling systems deserve the same scrutiny as any other advertisement.

Ecology and Ethics Labels

As conscientious consumers have become more aware of the relationship between food safety and the environment and increasingly alarmed about food contamination, over-fishing, clear-felled forests, loss of biodiversity, climate change, and other environmental and health-related risks of food production, we've seen an explosion in the numbers of different programs and schemes that attempt to assure us that products so labeled are made through sustainable agricultural practices or that their manufacturers demonstrate good social and environmental performance. The Certified Humane and the Fair Trade label are only two examples of these.

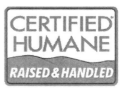

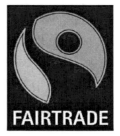

Many consumers want to take environmental and social ethics issues into account in their shopping, but recent research has shown that some of these labels have a "halo" effect on buyers. Foods that are perceived as having a high ethical value, e.g., the manufacturer provides its workers with good wages and health care, are also perceived as being nutritious or low calorie.[21]

It can be difficult to know which of these increasingly prevalent seals and labels can be trusted and what relationship they have, if any, to nutrition. As in the case of nutritional self-endorsement programs, these have to be evaluated on a case-by-case basis. A helpful Eco-label Decoder can be found on the Consumer Reports website.

Country of Origin Labels

In 2002, as part of the farm bill, congress included a mandatory Country of Origin Labeling (COOL) program intended to go into effect in September of 2004. Industry and trade objections delayed COOL implementation, but after a series of scandals over imported foods, regulation was finalized in 2009. An especially popular consumer policy, and a win on the labeling front in the Great American Food Fight, COOL requires retailers to declare where red meat, chicken, goat, fresh and frozen fruits and vegetables, peanuts, pecans, macadamia nuts, and ginseng was grown or harvested. Examples of COOL statements include: *Product of the U.S., Produce of the U.S., Grown in the U.S., or Country X.*

The supermarket industry and the World Trade Organization (WTO) are already calling for repeal of COOL legislation, citing the law as protectionist and unnecessary, but for now consumers have access to more information regarding the source of certain foods.

Expiration Dates

An expiration date, in some form, is another common element on the exterior of packaging. It is often an important consideration for purchase, and yet, contrary to the belief of most US consumers, there is currently no federal law that requires that expiration dates be published on anything but infant formula and baby food. Some states have their own regulations requiring freshness dating on dairy products and eggs, but beyond this, labeling is voluntary on the part of manufacturers.

Pictures and Graphics

The most powerful lure on the front of many packages is a beautiful depiction of the whole, fresh foods from which the product is presumably manufactured. While shoppers in a hurry are particularly vulnerable to the appeal of that colorful wholesomeness, there may be little or no relationship between those pretty pictures and what's actually inside the box. The U.S. Court of Appeals recently ruled against Gerber for using deceptive marketing techniques in the graphics used to decorate their Graduates Juice Treats for Toddlers. The package depicted a "medley" of fruits, including oranges, grapes, cherries, apples, raspberries and lemons. The main ingredients in the juice treats, however, are high fructose corn syrup and sugar. The only fruit there is nutritionally poor white grape juice concentrate. The court found that consumers should not be expected to look beyond misleading representations on the front of the box to discover the truth in the ingredient list in small print on the side of the box.

The labels of jellies, jams, and preserves are frequently adorned with pictures of fruits that don't represent the main ingredient inside. Fruit snacks and fruit drinks often mislead in the same way.

Poison Packaging

Finally, the packaging material itself must be a source of concern for individuals and for families. At least two potentially harmful chemicals—bisphenol A, or BPA, and the phthalate, DEHP, have been implicated in cancers, heart disease, and brain disorders. These chemicals are known to disrupt hormonal systems in the bodies of both animals and people, leading to developmental and reproductive problems. Both of them appear in a wide range of food packaging materials.

BPA

The history of BPA reads like a fiction thriller, containing elements of surprise, intrigue, political controversy and, some have suggested, even conspiracy. First synthesized in 1891, bisphenol A came into use as a synthetic estrogen in the 1930s. (Yes, a synthetic *estrogen.*) The shape and size of BPA allows it to fit into, and fool, the receptors in our bodies that recognize estrogen.

With the discovery in the 1960s that BPA could be combined with other compounds (like the toxic gas, phosgene) to produce stiff, shatter-resistant plastic, the chemical suddenly had new and almost unlimited potential. Since then it has been used to produce a host of products calling for a clear polycarbonate plastic. Headlights for cars, lenses for eyeglasses, and bottles for babies were a few of them. See-thru pet cages were another. That's where Patricia Hunt comes in.

In 1998, while working on genetics research at Washington State University, Hunt observed that control mice kept in polycarbonate cages had an unusually high number of chromosomally abnormal eggs. The lab's investigation revealed that a janitor had been scrubbing the cages, releasing bisphenol A into the animals' environment.

Hunt became a whistle-blower for the dangers of BPA and one of the world's leading researchers on aneuploidy, the error in cell division that causes spontaneous miscarriages and human birth defects, including Down syndrome. Her research inspired others to experiment with rat models and in the next years BPA was implicated in

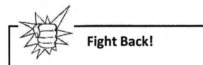

Fight Back!

Participate in one of the letter-writing campaigns to tell major food manufactures to get the BPA out of our foods. Get involved at **momsrising.org** or **breastcancerfund.org**

behavior disorders, heart disease, cancer, obesity, diabetes, and the prostate and neural development of fetuses, infants and children.

In 2006, the National Toxicology Program (NTP) looked at the growing body of evidence on BPA and pronounced the chemical safe, but the next year investigative journalists for the *Milwaukee Journal Sentinel* decided to take their own look. Their review of 258 studies found that the NTP had missed or selectively ignored many readily available studies which cited harm from BPA while including and giving extra weight to industry-funded studies. Even the financial consultant hired to compile the studies had financial ties to companies that made BPA.

In 2008, the FDA doubled down, declaring again that BPA was safe. But amid the outcry of health advocates and some lawmakers, and in light of additional research associating BPA exposure to cardiovascular disease, Type 2 diabetes, and liver enzyme abnormalities in adults, the FDA announced in 2009 that it would review 100 newer studies. In 2010, the agency reversed its earlier stance, citing "some concern" about the potential effects of BPA on the brain, behavior, and prostate gland in fetuses, infants, and young children, and promising to "take steps" to get BPA out of infant formula cans and baby bottles. While Canada, the European Union countries, Japan, China, and Malaysia have all imposed bans on BPA, its use is still legal in all US products.

There's good news in the fact that eleven states so far have issued their own bans on BPA, and many manufacturers of children's food and other products have voluntarily stopped using BPA in production. These actions, however, may not be not nearly enough. The Center for Disease Control and Prevention (CDC) has found that 93 percent of Americans have detectable levels of BPA by-products in their urine.[22] Even a BPA-free label may offer false comfort. When scientists conducted lab tests on more than 20 top-brand baby bottles as well as more than 450 plastic food and beverage-packages, virtually all of them leached chemicals that acted like the hormone estrogen, even though many claimed to be free of BPA.

As part of their *Cans not Cancer* campaign, the Breast Cancer Fund released two studies in late 2011 that found that BPA still appeared in a wide variety of canned foods specifically marketed to kids. Among these were Campbell's Disney Princess Cool Shapes Pasta with Chicken in Chicken Broth and Campbell's Toy Story Fun Shapes noodles. The Fund's study generated more than 70,000 letters to Campbell's, which has since promised to phase out BPA.

Clearly, consumers can influence manufacturers to produce foods without this dangerous chemical, but it appears that we'll have to continue the fight in this battle without government help. In March 2012, the FDA again rejected a ban on BPA

DEHP

DEHP (diethylhexylphthalate) is one of the phthalates, another class of endocrine-disrupting chemicals. Used since the 1930s as a softening agent, or plasticizer, it is ubiquitous in flexible vinyl products, cosmetics, perfumes, and other personal care products. Because DEHP is used in so many consumer products and is an unavoidable environmental contaminant, humans are exposed to DEHP at some level on a daily basis throughout life, from conception to death.

Animal studies have linked DEHP to inhibition of testosterone synthesis and adverse effects on the developing reproductive system of males. Some epidemiologic evidence also links urinary levels of phthalate metabolites to effects on boys' reproductive development, male hormone levels, and semen quality.

A major human exposure to phthalates is believed to be from foods which have absorbed the chemical from their packaging, but little research has been undertaken to verify this theory. One small study, however, seems to demonstrate that we can significantly reduce our levels of BPA and DEHP by choosing more whole, fresh foods over canned and packaged ones. In this study, five 4-person families were tested while eating their ordinary diets and again while eating a fresh food diet. When consuming their customary diets, family members' urine levels of both BPA and DEHP were in the range of the general U.S. population, as estimated by the CDC and Nutrition Examination

Survey program. During the time the families were on the fresh-food diet, concentration of BPA dropped by 66%, and concentrations of DEHP metabolites decreased by 53–56%.[23]

Food manufacturers and the makers of food storage plastics have begun to address consumer concerns about the dangers of these estrogenic chemicals. The Appendix provides a list of manufacturers who have pledged that their products are BPA-free.

Plastic Coding

We have some help in identifying dangerous plastics through the codes used to facilitate their recycling. These recycling codes, numbered 1 through 7, usually appear stamped on the bottoms of containers in an embossed triangle like this:

A chart explaining the types of plastics these codes describe and their associated dangers can be found in the Appendix. Use the codes to evaluate plastics you buy or have on hand.

Here are some additional steps you can take to reduce risks:

- Don't microwave plastic containers or any food in plastic cling wrap unless you're sure the plastic is BPA free.

- Wash recyclable bottles by hand. Don't scour polycarbonate plastic containers or put them in the dishwasher with harsh detergents.

- When possible, opt for glass, porcelain, or stainless steel containers, particularly for hot food or liquids.

- Since BPA is often used in the epoxy resin that lines the inside of cans, choose fresh or frozen foods for greatest risk reduction.

- Use infant formula bottles, dishes and sippy cups that are BPA free.

Eating in the Meantime

- Decisions about over-paying for over-packaging are personal and situational. Just keep in mind that there's an almost an inverse relationship between the prettiness and complexity of the package and the nutritional value of the food. A perfectly packaged food looks like a banana. Or a squash.

- Farmers markets and food co-ops are the best at minimizing packaging, but even in the supermarket we can make a difference by refraining from buying bagged or shrink-wrapped produce, by buying in bulk whenever possible, and taking our own recyclable grocery bags to shop.

- When you suspect slack fill, look at the net weight of the product you're considering and compare weights and box sizes of nearby products. To file a complaint, contact an FDA district complaint coordinator. A list of coordinators for each state can be found on the www.fda.gov website.

- Let the alarm bells go off when you notice new packaging for a familiar product. Be sure to check the price label to see if you're actually getting less.

- Develop a healthy scepticism about front-of-package labeling. We're all subject to self-deception, but we can get smarter. And always read the Nutrition Facts Panel.

- The names of many prepared meals or dishes are cultural hand-me-downs. We can't blame the manufacturer if we're surprised to discover there's no meat in a mincemeat pie or that Welsh rabbit is actually cheese toast. Imported or ethnic foods can be especially problematic in that they employ foreign language terms or have geographical references. They can, however, provide great learning opportunities for teaching kids about the many differences between what packages say and what's actually inside.

- Think through vacuous endorsement claims. "Recommended by the American Heart Association" may carry some weight, once you understand the way endorsements really work. But movie stars and athletes are rarely experts on nutrition. And claims like "Kid approved," "Doctor recommended," and "Preferred by Moms" are pure marketing hype.

- Don't confuse eco-labeling with organic labeling. And don't fall victim to the "halo effect" of social ethics labels. These labels don't tell us anything about nutrition.

- COOL labels are not identified graphically. They're text only, and you have to look for them. Ask your store manager if you have questions about country of origin.

- Replace water bottles that have been on the soccer field, and in the sun, too long. Whenever possible, choose plastics with the recycling code 1, 2 or 5. Recycling codes 3 and 7 are more likely to contain BPA or phthalates.

- Call or email the manufacturers of products that you must purchase in cans. Find out if can linings are BPA free.

- To reduce the risks of DEHP contamination, don't store or re-heat leftover pizza in its delivery box. To reduce BPA risks, transfer takeout foods from their original plastic containers to something safer before re-heating in the microwave.

- Vote on your grocery list ballot for poison-free packaging and those manufacturers who label their products truthfully.

Chapter 3. Bragging Up Front: Nutrition Claims on Packaging

We expect to find the health value of processed foods in that ruled box, the Nutrition Facts panel, on the back or side of the package. But the fronts of packages make claims about the product's nutritional value, too. These claims are often emblazoned in bright, bold lettering and they profoundly influence consumer choice. Research suggests that we put a lot of faith in these claims. Too much, perhaps. We frequently believe that front-of-package claims are government-endorsed, and we use them to ignore or override the Nutrition Facts Panel. The reality, however, is that all claims that appear on the front or sides of packaging are forms of advertising.

Who Decides What's Healthy?

To those of us accustomed to studying food labels—and to counting calories, fats, and carbs—the discovery that nutrition labeling is a relatively new development comes as something of a surprise. Many of us grew up before packages said anything at all about nutrition and for our parents even the marvel of the TV dinner was just "dinner." Nutrition food labeling was voluntary and unstandardized. We were pretty much on our own to decide whether or not it was healthy.

It wasn't until 1994 that the Nutrition Labeling and Education Act (NLEA) required packaged foods to bear nutrition labeling and demanded that all health claims for foods be "consistent with terms defined by the Secretary of Health and Human Services." The law, which had been vigorously opposed by food manufacturers, initiated the pitched battle between public health nutritionists and agribusiness and food processors that continues to this day. It has come to involve virtually every word or phrase that can appear on processed products and extends to their placement, their font size, even punctuation. It's a battle that overwhelms the resources of the FDA, but provides lucrative, lifelong careers for lobbyists and lawyers.

The Nutritional Standards Alphabet

The intent of the NLEA was to standardize nutrition information, but it didn't have to start from scratch to do it. Internationally recognized nutrition standards had existed since 1941 and been subsequently revised every five to ten years. We know these standards as RDAs, or Recommended Dietary Allowances.

RDAs

The original RDAs, sometimes also called the Recommended Daily Allowances, listed specific recommended intakes for calories and nine essential nutrients: protein, iron, calcium, vitamins A and D, thiamin, riboflavin, niacin, and vitamin C. The RDA recommendations suggested a daily dietary intake level sufficient to meet the nutrient requirements of nearly all (approximately 98 percent) healthy individuals.

DRIs

In 1997, six new nutrients (Vitamin K, Selenium, Chloride, Manganese, Chromium, and Molybdenum) were added to the RDA standards, as well as three more category definitions: The umbrella term for this broader, more detailed set of dietary guidelines, became Dietary Reference Intakes (DRI). The DRI is used to determine the recommended Daily Value (DVs) which are printed on food labels in the U.S. and Canada.

DRVs

The Daily Reference Values (DRV) are established for special components of foods not listed by the RDI's, such as Fat, Cholesterol, Carbohydrates, and Protein. Unlike other daily nutritional requirements, the DRV's are derived from how many calories a day you need.

It's important to remember that these are guidelines only, and very general ones at that. The three-month-old baby, the eighty-year-old woman, and the NFL linebacker have vastly different nutritional needs.

Core Nutrient Content Claims

There are eleven core terms that are regulated to some degree by the FDA. These are "free," "low," "lean," "extra lean," "high," "good source," "reduced," "less," "light," "fewer," and "more." Most of these apply in relation to the established or daily reference value (DRV) of a vitamin, mineral, fiber, or protein based on a 2,000-calorie diet for healthy adults.

The **less**, **fewer**, and **reduced** claims, for example, all mean that a product so advertised should have 25% less of a nutrient that the food it is referencing. These three are the easy ones, and the other end of the comparison spectrum isn't too complicated either. The **High** claim, and its synonym, **Excellent source of**, means that the food provides 20% more of the Daily Value for a given nutrient than the comparison food, while a **Good Source of*** food provides 10% of the Daily Value.

Here's the breakdown on these terms that make comparisons to the DRV:

Less, Fewer, or Reduced = 25% less

High*, Excellent, or Rich = 20% more

Good source*or More* (added, extra, plus) = 10% more

The **free from** claim, however, is more problematic. Current regulations allow food manufacturers to round down to zero any ingredient that accounts for less than 0.5 grams per serving. So, while a front of package label may claim that a product is "gluten-free" or "alcohol-free," or contains "No dangerous Trans fats," these ingredients will still appear listed on the back on the Nutrition Facts Panel. The "rounding down" loophole results in blatant falsehoods on front of package labels and illustrates one of the many reasons why consumers find label reading so confusing.

In addition to these core terms, and the multitude of synonyms for them, there are other words and phrases commonly used on front of package labeling to entice us to buy and to convince us of the safety or nutritional value of various products. Our list is by no means exhaustive but is meant to highlight the terms that are most misinterpreted by consumers. Regulated terms are marked with an asterisk. The others, while they may imply health or nutritional benefits are just, well, words.

Enriched and Fortified Claims

The terms **enriched** and **fortified** often grab our attention on packaging and subsequently grab our grocery dollar. Many consumers believe these terms are equivalent and that both simply mean they're getting "extra" vitamins or nutrients. When it comes to fortified foods that may actually be the case. **Fortification** refers to the practice of deliberately increasing the content of vitamins and minerals in a food regardless of whether the nutrients were originally present in the food before processing. **Enriched** means that the manufacturer has artificially added back nutrients that were lost in processing. A food that is labeled as "enriched" with a nutrient must contain at least 10 percent more of the Daily Value of that nutrient than a food of the same type that is not enriched.

There's nothing new about the idea of adding vitamins and minerals to foods. The discovery that iodine reduced the prevalence of goiter led to its inclusion in salt in the 20s. Milk has been fortified with Vitamin D since the 40s and its addition helped to eliminate rickets. Flour and rice are routinely enriched with niacin, thiamin, riboflavin and iron to restore nutrients lost in the milling of these grains. In 1998, the U.S. Food and Drug Administration made it mandatory to include folic acid in enriched grains such as breads and cereals with the goal of reducing neural-tube defects in infants. What *is* rather new in terms of food production is the idea of prescriptive or functional foods—foods that can treat or eliminate health problems.

Functional Foods

The line between food and medicine has blurred considerably in the last two decades. Today our grocery aisles are flooded with foods that promise health benefits far beyond their basic nutritional value. These benefits range from memory lapses cured by herbs, to digestive disturbances cured by beneficial bacteria (probiotics), to heart attacks prevented by plant sterols. In between there are thousands of products that claim to promote health or prevent disease.

The market for these so-called "functional foods" has become one of the fastest growing industries in the US. Already a multi-billion dollar industry, experts predict annual growth rates of 7% or higher for the functional food market, but no one dares predict how far this new wave may carry us. The red wine "pill" has already been developed, and some researchers already foresee the day of edible vaccines.

While the trend is certainly good for the financial health of processed food manufacturers, environmentalists and health policy experts worry that the clamor for functional additives may be providing a slippery slope for more genetically modified foods. Nutritionists and scientists also see hazards for the consumer that may outweigh the benefits. Chief among them is simple safety.

Regulatory authorities around the world tend to be years behind the companies introducing these products. Our own FDA requires nutrition facts only for those substances with FDA daily values, such as vitamin A or calcium. Amounts of ingredients such as Omega-3 fatty acid and probiotics are not regulated. Consumers can't know how much they should be ingesting because manufacturers are not required to disclose how much or little they are putting in their foods.

Another concern is the possibility of overdose, or *hyper-vitaminosis*. The combination of taking multivitamins while also consuming fortified nutrition bars, health drinks and cereals may be too much of a good thing. Vitamin A, for example, is vital at low doses, but may be toxic at levels only 10 times those required to prevent deficiencies. Studies have suggested that long-term intake of a diet high in vitamin A may promote the development of osteoporotic hip fractures in women.[24] The Harvard School of Public Health (HSPH) has also warned about consuming too much folic acid from food.

The HSPH doesn't suggest we give up our daily multivitamin-multi-mineral supplement, but that we avoid heavily fortified foods that deliver a full day's dose—or sometimes more—of folic acid [25]

> The combination of taking multivitamins while also consuming fortified nutrition bars, health drinks and cereals may be too much of a good thing.

The biggest worry, however, is that these new prescription foods might encourage consumers to switch from a diverse, healthy diet to a basically unhealthy one – with an increasing reliance on functional additives or modifications. The front package claim, "Fortified with essential vitamins and minerals," on products like breakfast cereal and drinks can be a powerful distraction from the fact that these products often contain high amounts of sugar.

While enriched or fortified foods can make significant contribution to nutrient intakes, they do not have the same nutritional benefits as the whole foods for which they substitute. The whole food will always be superior.

Calorie Claims

With the exception of certain foods that have been engineered to be calorie free, like artificial sugar substitutes, there are no negative calorie foods. The FDA, however, allows the misleading claim of

Calorie Free* on products that contain fewer than 5 calories per serving. **Zero Calories, No Calories, Without Calories, Trivial Source of Calories,** and **Negligible Source of Calories** are other variants on the calorie free claim. Serving sizes are often manipulated in order to make these claims and, of course, many of us consume more than one serving.

Many whole foods are extremely low in calories. Celery, for example, has been touted as a perfect food, in that more calories are burned in eating and digesting it than are initially present in the food. Practically speaking, however, we can't eat sufficient quantities of celery, or apples, or cucumbers, to trick our bodies into calorie deficits.

Low Calorie, or Lo Cal* are regulated claims meaning that each serving supplies 40 or fewer calories. **Reduced calorie*** indicates at least 25 percent fewer calories per serving than the comparison food.

Carbohydrate Claims

The FDA has never defined carbohydrate claims and thus the use of terms like "low-carb," "reduced carb" or "carb free" is illegal. In the absence of regulatory guidelines, many food manufacturers have created their own terminology for carbohydrate content. Expressions like "net carbs," "impact carbs," or "effective carbs" emblazon food packages, but have no legal or scientific definition. Some brands make implied low-carbohydrate claims with phrases like "carb smart," "carb aware," and "carb sense."

Both the Grocery Manufacturers Association and the CSPI have called upon the FDA to set standards for labeling low carb products, but, for now, consumers are on their own. Carbohydrate claims are meaningless.

Cholesterol Claims

Cholesterol free*, or **No cholesterol*** generally means that the product contains less than 2 milligrams per serving. **Low cholesterol*** means 20 milligrams or less per serving and 2 grams or less of saturated fat per serving.

Cholesterol is only found in animal products, but you will still find "cholesterol free" claims on products that contain no animal components. Specific cholesterol-lowering claims can only be made legally for drugs, but the FDA is a little slow to catch up. The Cheerios box claimed to "lower your cholesterol 4% in six weeks" for more than two years.

Fat Claims

Fat Free* – A fat free product contains a half-gram of fat or less per serving. In a **Low Saturated Fat*** product, one gram or less per portion is saturated fat.

Low Fat* – A low fat product contains 3 grams of fat or less per serving. **Contains a Small Amount of Fat** and **Less Fat** are synonyms, but **Less fat** claims are usually specific and compare fat content to an original version of the product. A claim of "33% less fat" may be accurate in the comparison, but the decreased fat may be offset by additional carbohydrates in the form of refined flour or sugar to keep the product palatable.

Lite, light* – When this claim applies to fat it means that the food has at least 50% less fat or 1/3 fewer calories per serving than the "regular" full-fat food cited on the label. "Light" may also be used to indicate properties of texture or color, like light olive oil, or light brown sugar.

Lean* – In a 3-ounce portion of meat, seafood, poultry or game meat labeled as lean, there must be fewer than 10 grams of total fat, fewer than 4.5 grams saturated fat, and no more than 95 milligrams of cholesterol. **Extra Lean*** means that the food contains fewer than 5 grams of total fat, fewer than 2 grams of saturated fat, and no more than 95 milligrams cholesterol per three ounces.

No Trans fats, Contains 0 grams of Trans-fats, and zero Trans fats*claims mean that labeled foods have less than .5 grams of Trans fats per serving, not that they have no Trans fats. A quick check of the Nutrition Facts panel often reveals hydrogenated oils among the list of ingredients.

Fiber Claims

The FDA requires dietary fiber to be included on the Nutrition Facts Panel and yet has no written definition of even what constitutes "fiber." This omission allows manufacturers to add isolated fibers to a variety of unlikely foods like ice creams, yogurts, juices and drinks so that they can brag about their fiber content." In its *Food Labeling Chaos Report*, the Center for Science in the Public Interest illustrates this point with General Mills Fiber One Chew Bars, and their "35% Daily Value of Fiber" front of pack claim. The fiber, however, comes from Chicory Root Extract.[26]

The approved fiber claims are

More or added Fiber* – A portion of this food serves 2.5 grams of fiber

Good Source of Fiber* – A serving with this claim contains 2.5 to 4.9 grams of fiber.

High Fiber* – A portion of this food serves at least 5 grams of dietary fiber.

For now, however, these fibers may come from purified powders like inulin, polydextrose and maltodextrin, even cellulose, rather than the intact fibers found in whole foods and associated with health benefits.

Freshness Claims

We assume that "fresh" foods have the most nutritional potency, but freshness claims are more problematic than valuable.

Fresh*– The term "fresh," means that the food is unprocessed, in its raw state, and has not been frozen or subjected to any form of thermal processing or other preservation.

Fresh frozen, frozen fresh*– These terms mean that a food has been recently harvested before freezing, while **quickly frozen*** means frozen by a specific freezing system such as blast freezing.

For added freshness indicates that a chemical preservative has been added to prolong shelf life. BHA and BHT (Butylated hydroxyanisole and Butylated hydroxytoluene) are widely used to preserve freshness. (See Chapter 6 for a discussion of these food additives.)

Use of any of these freshness claims does not preclude the food from having been waxed or coated, from the post-harvest use of approved pesticides, from the application of a mild chlorine wash or acid wash on produce, or the treatment of raw foods with ionizing radiation.

Many lines of fruit juices and tomato sauces carry the word "fresh" on the label but are actually reconstituted from industrial concentrate.

Grain Claims

Multigrain, seven grain, whole grain, whole wheat – Bread, pasta, crackers, waffles, and similar baked products with these labels may indeed contain whole, or many, grains while still being largely composed of refined white flour and stripped of essential nutrients. The only way to know for sure is to turn the box over to read the Nutrition Facts Panel. In its 2010, *Food Labeling Chaos Report*, The CSPI recommended to the FDA that the "Made with whole wheat" claim be accompanied by a statement disclosing what percentage of total grains in the product are whole. Presently, many products making such claims are still made primarily from ordinary wheat flour.

Natural Claims

All natural, natural, made with natural ingredients – While many shoppers assume that a product advertised as natural is exceptionally wholesome or nutritious, this favorite claim of food marketers is almost meaningless. In the United States, neither the FDA (which discourages its use) nor the Department of Agriculture has any standards at all which apply to the use of labeling foods as "natural." In its published collection of international standards, the *Codex Alimentarius*, the Food and Agriculture Organization of the United Nations, doesn't even recognize the term. The single exception to current regulation of the term concerns natural flavors. The FDA defines a natural flavor as one derived "from a spice, fruit or fruit juice, vegetable or vegetable juice, edible yeast, herb, bark, bud, root, leaf" or similar plant (or even animal) material. Unfortunately, as of this writing, manufacturers are not required to tell us which "natural" spice, fruit, etc., is involved.

Several different class action law suits have been filed over use of the "natural" term. ConAgra has been challenged because its Wesson Oil products contain genetically modified organisms (GMOs). In a similar suit against Frito-Lay, plaintiffs contend that marketing describing products in the Tostitos and SunChips lines as "all natural" are made of genetically modified ingredients. In 2011 the Kellogg Company was sued over its "all natural" Kashi brand products which plaintiffs claimed contain "a spectacular array of unnaturally processed and synthetic ingredients." As part of the class action settlement Kellogg agreed to drop the "all natural" and "nothing artificial" terms from products in its Kashi line. A 2012 lawsuit against Tropicana alleges that its "100% pure and natural" claim on orange juice is fraudulent. The lawsuit claims that Tropicana puts the juice through extensive processing, adding aromas, flavors, and additives to prolong shelf life.

Not all of these "natural" lawsuits even make it to trial, but the number of suits challenging use of the term on packaged foods has exploded in the last few years.

Organic Claims

As part of the 1990 Farm Bill, the USDA's National Organic Program (NOP) regulates the standards for any farm, wild crop harvesting, or handling operation that wants to sell an agricultural product as organically produced. The USDA maintains a National List of Allowed and Prohibited Substances that may and may not be used in organic crop and livestock production. Organic farmers are also required to adhere to certain soil and water conservation methods and to rules about the humane treatment of animals. Consumers buying organic products can also be assured that the foods are produced without antibiotics, hormones, pesticides, irradiation or bioengineering. Certification is handled by state, non-profit and private agencies that have been approved by the USDA.

There are actually <u>three</u> designations, or tiers, possible on an organically labeled product:

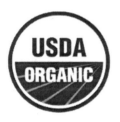

100% Organic* – According to the USDA's national organic standard, products labeled as "100 percent organic" must contain (excluding water and salt) only organically produced ingredients and processing aids. They should contain no chemicals, additives, synthetics, pesticides or genetically engineered substances and must also show an ingredient list and the name and address of the handler (bottler, distributor, importer, manufacturer, packer, processor, etc.). These products can display the USDA Organic logo and the logo of the certifying agent.

Organic* – To be labeled as "organic," 95% of the ingredients must be organically grown and the remaining 5% must come from non-organic ingredients that have been approved on the National List. These products can also display the USDA organic logo and the certifier's logo.

Made With Organic Ingredients – Food products labeled as "made with organic ingredients" must be made with at least 70% organic ingredients, three of which must be listed on the back of the package and again, the remaining 30% of the non-organic ingredients must approved on the National List. These products may display the certifier's logo, but not the USDA organic logo.

Products containing less than 70 percent organic ingredients cannot use the word "organic" on the packaging or display panel, and the only place an organic claim can be made is on the ingredient label.

It's clear that consumers are confused about organic and "natural" labels on foods, too often believing that "natural" claims imply the absence of pesticides and genetically engineered organisms. Recent public opinion poll results, conducted by various research firms, confirm this, and food manufacturers intentionally use marketing techniques that exploit this confusion. Those producers and distributors who conform to organic standards are concerned that misleading and ill-defined "natural" labeling is undermining the authentic Organic label.

Antibiotic free, hormone free and similar claims are not backed by any certifying organization. **Raised without added Hormones** is deliberately misleading when it appears on pork or poultry products as federal law prohibits the introduction of hormones to hogs and poultry.

Salt Claims

Sodium Free* – In a sodium free product, a single serving should provide fewer than 5 milligrams of sodium. **Lo Sodium**, or **Low Sodium** means that a portion contains 140 milligrams or less of sodium per serving, while **Very low-sodium** indicates that a product contains 35 mg sodium or less per serving.

Reduced sodium or **less sodium** indicates that a product contains at least 25% less sodium than the standard version. Some "reduced sodium" products, however, are still very high in sodium. For example, "reduced sodium" canned soups, though considerably lower in salt than regular canned soups, can still contain almost 500 milligrams sodium per 1-cup serving. "Light" or "lite" soy sauce, though considerably lower in salt than regular soy sauce, still contains 500-600 mg sodium per tablespoon. All front of pack claims should be taken with a grain of salt.

Light in sodium* indicates that the product contains at least 50% less sodium than the standard version. Note: Some "light in sodium" products are still very high in sodium, so you'll need to check the actual sodium content on the Nutrition Facts Panel to see if it fits into your low-sodium diet.

Unsalted or **No salt added** indicates that no additional sodium has been added during processing, but the product will still contain the sodium that naturally occurs in the product's ingredients.

Sugar Claims

Bragging about low or reduced sugar content helps to sell processed foods, but the range of sugar claims can be highly confusing. The **No sugar added*** claim is increasingly taking a prominent position on front of package labeling and consumers often believe that the label means a sugarless, or at least a low sugar product. In fact the claim often appears on products naturally high in sugars. The "no sugar added" claim only means that no sugar has been added *beyond* that which naturally occurs in the food. The product may still contain sweeteners and simple carbohydrates like turbinado, dextrose, honey, maltose, sucrose, fructose, corn syrup, or lactose, all of which contain calories and contribute to weight gain.

The phrases **lightly sweetened** or **Low sugar** are good for sales, too, and are most likely to appear on cereal packages. While the FDA regulates the use of "sugar free" and "no added sugars," it does not govern claims of "low sugar" or "lightly sweetened." The CSPI thinks that the decisions like whether "Kellogg's Frosted Mini-Wheats Bite Size" is lightly sweetened should be determined by federal rules, not the marketing executives of a manufacturer. [26]

Reduced Sugar and **Less sugar** claims signify that the product has at least 25% less sugar than an appropriate reference food. For example, a chocolate ice cream would use as its reference food, other chocolate ice creams. A food that is not actually low in calories but bears a claim regarding the absence of sugar must be accompanied, each time it is used, by one of the following disclaimer statements:

"not a reduced calorie food," "not a low calorie food," or "not for weight control."

Sugar free*, no sugar, zero sugar, and similar claims do not necessarily mean the absence of sugar. These claims may be legally printed on a food's label if it contains fewer than 0.5 grams of sugar per serving, so checking serving size is critical to determining how much sugar you're actually ingesting. These claims commonly appear on diabetic-friendly foods, fruit-flavored waters, and diet sodas. Sugar-free beverages may still contain artificial sweeteners like Splenda or Aspartame. See Chapter 10 for an extensive discussion of sugar and artificial sweeteners.

Dietary Guidance Symbols

The first government *Dietary Guidelines for Americans* was issued in 1980 and has been jointly published by the Departments of Agriculture (USDA) and Health and Human Services (HHS) every five years since, with the most recent issue coming in 2010.

A series of symbols, often appearing on food packaging, has accompanied evolving dietary guidance over the years. Beginning in 1943, we had The Basic 7, followed by the Basic Four (1956–1992), the Food Guide Pyramid (1992–2005), and My Pyramid (2005–2011). In June, 2011, The My Pyramid logo was supplanted by MyPlate, (shown in Chapter 1) which depicts a suggested ratio from five food groups. MyPlate was widely received as an improvement on the My Pyramid icon, which had been criticized as too abstract and confusing. The greater emphasis on fruits and vegetables, as well as the simplicity and clarity of the plate image, has been particularly praised.

Some critics, however, see MyPlate as the mere shuffling of deckchairs on the Titanic. Complaints, to name only a few, include the fact that the new image puts undue emphasis on milk and meat, doesn't distinguish between whole and refined grains, and doesn't encourage a variety of fruits and vegetables.

In response to these objections The Harvard School of Public Health released its own adjusted and more detailed version of

MyPlate, called the Harvard Healthy Eating Plate. Harvard's plate features a higher ratio of vegetables to fruit, adds healthy oils to the recommendation, and balances healthy protein and whole grains as equal quarters of the plate, along with recommending water while limiting dairy consumption. The Harvard plate also contains a recommendation for physical activity.

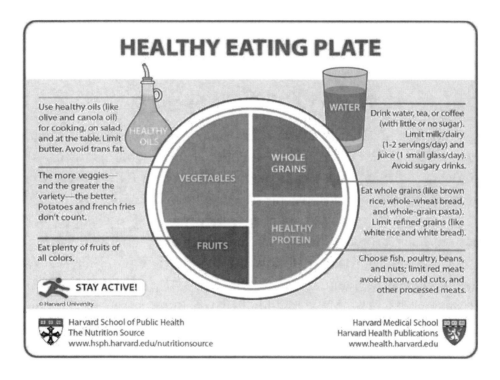

Shelf-Tag Labels

One of the newest food labeling systems attempts to catch the consumer eye not on the front of the package, but on the front of the shelf. Shelf tag label systems are managed by grocery chains and give foods a nutritional grade or score. The *Nuval* system gives a numerical score based on several factors associated with the food (1 to 100, with 100 being best). The *Guiding Stars* system awards one to three stars.

Safeway has initiated SimpleNutrition, which uses 22 different benefit tags. Wal-Mart's *Great for You* system is meant to identify items that meet the government's 2010 Dietary Guidelines. Several regional grocery chains have also initiated their own systems.

Critics of these shelf-tag labeling systems say they simply add clutter to an already confusing label landscape and believe that only objective third parties without financial interests should be grading foods.

Guiding Stars

The Future of Food Labeling

In 2010, First Lady Michelle Obama challenged the food industry to develop a front-of-pack labeling system that could be widely adopted on food packages and that would help busy consumers—especially parents—make more informed decisions when they shop. In response, the CDC and the FDA commissioned an objective body, The Institute of Medicine (IOM), to convene an expert committee to issue recommendations for front-of-package labeling. In the meantime, however, The Grocery Manufacturers of America and the Food Marketing Institute joined forces to develop and implement the Nutrition Keys initiative, a labeling system that will put nutrition information on the front of food and beverage packages. Four basic icons represent calories, along with saturated fat, sodium and sugars—the nutrients which dietary guidance recommends limiting. The label also may also include up to two other nutrients, such as

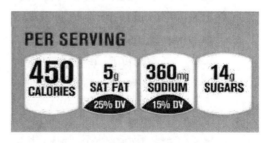

potassium, fiber, vitamin A, vitamin C, vitamin D, calcium, iron and protein. Consumers should start seeing the icons in supermarkets next year.

Not everyone is on board with the Nutrition Keys program. Some critics say the industry is trying a pre-emptive strike to avoid using the plan being developed by the FDA. Kelly Brownell, Director of the Rudd Center for Food Policy and Obesity at Yale, thinks the new labels are an abuse of trust by the food industry and an effort to "lock in a system that would change food choices as little as possible and preempt the imposition of an alternative system that would be based on the available relevant science."[27]

Until the government exercises its authority to mandate science-based nutrition labeling, everything on the front of all those pretty packages means the buyer must beware.

While the new program may be a step in the right direction, it's unlikely that a public health objective will ever be the primary goal of a food industry-based labeling system. Until the government exercises its authority to mandate science-based nutrition labeling, everything on the front of all those pretty packages means the buyer must beware.

Eating in the Meantime

- Products labeled reduced-fat are not necessarily better choices than the regular versions. More sugar and sodium are often added to make up for the lower fat content. Read the nutrition facts panel, as many reduced fat brands will contain Trans fatty acids or partially hydrogenated oils. *See Chapter 5, The Big Fat Lies about Fat.*

- It may be comforting to find the term "natural," printed on the processed foods we buy, but we need to keep reminding ourselves that the term is all but meaningless. Individual companies determine their own set of "natural" standards, without public input, third-party certification, or government oversight.

- The less and reduced claims are meaningless without consulting the Nutrition Facts panel since the original product to which these claims refer may actually be high in fat, sugar, sodium or calories.

- A front of packaging notice to *See Nutrition Facts for* [content] is a sure giveaway. The product will usually be higher than the recommended suggestions for fat, saturated fat, cholesterol, or sugar.

- *Fresh* is often used in a number of phrases that may have an emotional appeal, but no real meaning. *Oven fresh, farm fresh, garden fresh, kitchen fresh, ocean fresh*, etc., are all examples. Many lines of fruit juices and tomato sauces also carry the word "fresh" on the label but are actually reconstituted from industrial concentrate.

- Product dating has recently become a marketing device for some manufactures who would like us to throw out and replace products that really can't expire, like soft drinks. Don't be intimidated. There's not much to expire with a beverage made of water, sugar, and artificial coloring.

- All shelf tag labeling systems are proprietary. If you shop several stores, the nutritional criteria will vary. And don't expect to find tags that warn you to avoid particular foods. Nutrition information is the secondary goal of these systems.

- **Enriched** and **fortified** are not synonyms for healthy. Remember that added vitamins and minerals in processed foods don't affect the high amount of sugar that is present or necessarily make the product healthy. Don't be seduced into buying a processed food for its "added" vitamins or antioxidants alone. The best source of all nutrients is still a balanced diet based on whole, natural foods.

- Producers who sell less than $5,000 a year in organic foods are exempt from USDA certification. The small producer or farmer may still follow the USDA's standards for organic foods.

- Always keep in mind that manufacturers optimize labeling for sales, not health.

- We all know it, but we forget. The most nutritious foods in the supermarket are the least packaged. Shopping the perimeter of the store will buy you the most nutrition for your shopping dollar.

Chapter 4. Food Additives: Subtracting from your Family's Health

Direct food additives are used for the purpose of extending shelf life, enhancing appearance or texture, increasing or altering flavor, adding nutritional content, balancing acids, and more. The vast majority of the substances added to our food are synthetic compounds. They are perfectly legal (at least here in the US), and, as many will argue, the presence of almost any one of them in a single food product is minimal. Even where scientists turn up toxicity or carcinogenic effects in test studies, it's not an occasion for unnecessary concern. The laboratory tests that evaluate the risk of additives, where they've been undertaken, are usually conducted on mice or rats. People, of course, aren't rodents. And the dosages that are administered under test conditions are much greater—astronomically greater, we're told—than what any individual human would ever ingest. The "risk is minimal" argument is a good one. It allows the manufactures of these additives, and the food processors that incorporate them into the products we buy, a great deal of leeway, and a lot of time, for the jury to stay out.

The argument, however, doesn't take into account a great many factors that have enormous implications for the health of our individual families and even for our progeny. In scarcely more than a generation, we've gone from eating almost none of these synthetic ingredients to consuming many, and on a daily basis.

Here are just a few counterpoints to the "risk is minimal" argument:

- No one knows how many additives that the average adult, or the average child, consumes in a single meal or a single day, let alone in a whole year. The International Food Additives Council, a trade association which represents additive manufacturers, estimates that the consumption of food additives other than sugar and salt, but including black pepper, yeast, baking soda, citric acid, and mustard, would be about 14 pounds per year, or a little over half an ounce per day.

- We know almost nothing about the cumulative effects of these compounds. (No one today is willing to argue that cigarette smoking doesn't lead to cancer, or to say that the risk is minimal because the effects can take decades to show themselves.)

- We are largely ignorant of the synergistic effects of even the most commonly used additives. (What happens when X is combined with Y? When XY is added to Z?)

- We know little about how these additives change or are altered during cooking or processing. (Is X still safe after heating? Does Y change in the presence of X?)

- We know little about how cultural or socioeconomic factors affect our intake of particular additives. (Do Latin American families, for example, consume too much of particular additives because of their preference for certain foods?)

- We know little about susceptibilities to harm depending on individuals' life stage (for example, pregnant women, infants, children, and the elderly).

- We don't know how many food additives interact with chemicals in our environment or in common cosmetics or drugs.

Many of these issues are being addressed. They are being slowly and steadily explored in private, government, and university laboratories all over the world. In the meantime, more than 10,000 substances can be directly added to our foods for a myriad of reasons. There are no serious discussions underway about capping the list of additives in the interests of national health. There is certainly no financial incentive for manufacturers to agree to a ceiling. Globally, the market for additives is expected to reach more than $33 billion by 2015. And you can be sure that for every scientist working to investigate the safety of any single food additive, there are ten others, employed by monolithic food corporations, working to create another.

Among the many troubling aspects of additive proliferation is the obscurity of their chemical or scientific names and their mysterious purposes in our food. Our grandmothers baked bread with flour, eggs, yeast and water. Our own bread contains ingredients like sodium stearoyl lactate, potassium bromate, calcium propionate, mono and diglycerides, Butylated Hydroxy-anisole, and azodicarbonamide. And that's to name only a few. The iconic Twinkie, essentially a bread product, contains 39 ingredients, including mysterious-sounding components like *diacetyl* and *Polysorbate 60*. Must we all become part-time chemists to know what we're feeding our families? Increasingly, it seems that we must.

Who's Minding the Chemical Store?

The first law written to protect the public from adulterated or poisonous food and medicines was the Meat Inspection Act of 1906, which established federal inspection of meat products. The original Food and Drugs Act was passed by Congress on the same day. The Food and Drug Act forbade the manufacture, sale, or transportation of adulterated or misbranded food and medicines, and established what would become the FDA.

While it seems absurd to us today that anyone could oppose laws prohibiting poison or filth in our food, even these first protections didn't come easily. The patent medicine makers and their lobbies were extremely powerful and very well-funded. Representatives of the "beef trust" and other food producers vigorously fought the legislation and some members of Congress, particularly a number of Southern senators, opposed the bill on constitutional grounds.

Eventual enactment of these laws, under a sympathetic Theodore Roosevelt, came about only as a result of consumer outcry. The public had been horrified by slaughterhouse practices described in Upton Sinclair's novel, *The Jungle*. Samuel Hopkins Adams had garnered attention with sensational exposés of the patent medicine industry. Scientific support came from Dr. Harvey W. Wiley, the Department of Agriculture's chief chemist, who published his findings on the widespread use of harmful preservatives.

During the Great Depression, the Wheeler-Lea Act was passed to make false or misleading statements about foods, drugs and cosmetics illegal through product markings or advertising in interstate commerce. The Federal Trade Commission was given responsibility for the advertising portion and the Food and Drug Administration took charge of the misbranding issues.

The 1958 Food Additives Amendment to the Federal Food, Drug, and Cosmetic Act provided for the first specific regulations of food additives. In the years before its passage, the burden for proving the health dangers of any new additive fell to the government, but the 1958 amendment turned that on its head, shifting the responsibility to the manufacturer for proving the safety of any new additive. The Delaney Clause made the 1958 law tightened the law slightly by prohibiting the approval of any food additive shown to induce cancer in humans or animals. The food and chemical industries have sought to weaken or repeal the law since its passage.

Under the Food Additives Amendment, two groups of ingredients were exempted from the regulation process.

GROUP I - Prior-sanctioned substances are those that the FDA or USDA had determined safe for use in food prior to the 1958 amendment. Examples are sodium nitrite and potassium nitrite used to preserve luncheon meats. I'll have a lot to say about the harmful effects of these additives in Chapter 5, but nitrates are worth mentioning here because of the prevalence of their use today, not as a preservative, but as a coloring in hotdogs.

GROUP II - GRAS (generally recognized as safe) ingredients - are those that are generally recognized by experts as safe, based on their extensive history of use in food before 1958 or based on published scientific evidence. They do not require a pre-market review or approval process. Among the several hundred GRAS substances are salt, sugar, spices, vitamins, but also monosodium glutamate (MSG).

Other exclusions from the regulation included dietary supplements, drugs in animal feed, color additives, and certain pesticides.

How Do We Know It's Safe?

The simple answer is, we don't. Under our present system new additives are tested by the manufacturer rather than by an independent, third-party research organization with no stake in the industry or its regulation. The FDA has no way of acquiring complete information about the use of a substance in foods after it has been approved. Under the GRAS process, substances can be added to food even without the FDA's awareness and without the agency having access to the substance's use or safety data. Finally, the processes for both effecting and revoking food additive approvals are legalistic and cumbersome, which reduces the flexibility for public health decision making.

For many consumers, especially parents, the question of "What are they doing to our food?" is almost too overwhelming to consider. Many of us take the "ostrich" stance, just sticking our heads in the sand, hoping that tomorrow's headline news doesn't reveal that something that our children have been eating all their lives contributes to chronic disease, cancer, or infertility. We don't, however, need to live in a frenzy of fear. There are some steps we can take. Primarily we need to become conscientious label-readers, educating ourselves especially about those additives that may pose particular risk to susceptible family members, to children, or in pregnancy. The best approach, of course, is to eliminate processed foods to the greatest extent possible.

Additives under Suspicion

A full list of food additives is obviously impossible here. Most households would do well to keep a list of questionable additives in their wallets or tacked up near the pantry. Mobile technologies have also enabled shoppers to research chemical additives at the point of purchase. What follows below is a high-level review of those additives that are controversial, have been banned in other countries or in some US states, have been deemed human carcinogens, or are associated with known health risks. This discussion excludes caffeine, properly an additive but not regulated. It also omits artificial sweeteners, discussed at length in Chapter 10, and nitrate and nitrate meat additives taken up in Chapter 6.

Azodicarbonamide

A synthetic yellow-orange dough conditioner and flour bleacher, azodicarbonamide frequently appears in commercial bread products. It is also commonly used in the production of industrial foam plastic. Although the FDA has approved its use for food in the States, the United Kingdom, other European countries, and Australia has banned it as a potential cause of asthma. The use of azodicarbonamide in Singapore carries penalties of imprisonment and fine.

In a review of 47 studies on azodicarbonamide, the World Health Organization concluded that it probably does trigger asthmatic symptoms. The WHO advised that "exposure levels should be reduced as much as possible."[28] .

Many fast food chains use azodicarbonamide in bread and sandwich buns. Ask to see ingredient lists if you have susceptible family members.

Benzoic Acid, Sodium Benzoate

A preservative added to fruit juice, carbonated drinks, and pickles, sodium benzoate can create problems when used in beverages that also contain ascorbic acid (vitamin C). The two substances, in an acidic solution, can react together to form small amounts of benzene, a chemical that causes leukemia and other cancers. In the early 1990s the FDA urged companies not to use benzoate in products that also contain ascorbic acid, but companies are still using that combination. A lawsuit filed in 2006 by private attorneys ultimately forced Coca-Cola, PepsiCo, and other soft-drink makers in the U.S. to reformulate affected beverages, typically fruit-flavored products.

A 2007 study published in *The Lancet* found that a mixture of sodium benzoate and food dyes was linked to hyperactive behavior in children, although it was not clear whether the dyes or the preservative were to blame. [29] Since soft drinks are the main source of sodium benzoate in children's diets, parents have another good reason to limit cola consumption.

Butylated Hydroxyanisole (BHA)

An extremely common preservative used to retard the rancidity of fats and oils, BHA can be found in a multitude of products including cereals, chewing gum, potato chips, and vegetable oils. Studies demonstrating that BHA causes cancer in laboratory animals led the World Health Organization, in 1993, to recommend its removal from all foods, and it has since been banned in the European Union countries, in Canada, Nigeria, Brazil, Peru, Sri Lanka, Greece, Japan and China. According to the U.S. Toxicology Program, BHA is "reasonably anticipated to be a human carcinogen." The FDA still has approved the use of BHA as a food additive.

Butylated Hydroxytoluene (BHT)

Patented in 1947 and approved for use as a food additive and preservative in 1954, BHT is one of the most common GRAS additives used to keep fats and oils from going rancid. It is commonly used in cereals, chewing gum, vegetable oil and potato chips and in some food packaging to preserve freshness.

Controversy swirls around BHT, which has been linked in some studies to a potential increase in cancer, and in others to a decrease. There is evidence that some people may have difficulty metabolizing BHT, resulting in health and behavior changes, including child hyperactivity.

Fortunately, not all manufacturers use this preservative. Careful label reading can help you avoid it.

Calcium Propionate

Many consumers have concerns about this additive because of its almost ubiquitous presence in commercial bread products. Used to prevent mold and bacterial growth, it is the most commonly used preservative. While there is anecdotal evidence that calcium propionate causes MSG-like headaches for some sensitive individuals, there is no medical evidence to explain or support this claim. To date the accumulated research indicates that calcium propionate is non-toxic and safe to use in the amounts typically used by food manufacturers.

Carrageenan

While you may think that you don't normally eat seaweed, you probably do. Probably often. And in a surprising variety of foods. Carrageenan is a fiber extracted from red seaweed. Like cellulose (which also appears in processed food), it's indigestible to humans, but it works wonders when used as a thickening or gelling agent or as an emulsifier to keep ingredients in food from separating.

Start reading those labels and you'll notice that Carrageenan shows up everywhere. It's injected into raw chicken and other meats to help them retain water. It's used to keep cocoa from separating from milk in chocolate milk. It appears in ice creams, jellies, cottage cheese, toothpaste, fruit gushers, infant formulas and much, much more. It's even used to de-ice frozen airplanes.

Carrageenan was placed on the FDA list as a GRAS (generally recognized as safe) additive in the 1950s and grandfathered into the system with the 1958 Food Additives amendment as a prior sanctioned substance. Since carrageenan, like wood pulp, cannot be absorbed by the human stomach, there's a temptation to wonder how it even qualifies as "food," but leaving that aside, the additive's widespread use in our industrialized food supply is calling that dusty old safety status into question.

Some consumers complain of tummy aches after ingesting the additive and the science seems to be confirming that it has harmful effects on human intestinal cells. The consumption of carrageenan may have a role in intestinal inflammation and possibly in inflammatory bowel disease. In laboratory animals it's been shown to cause cancer and ulcerative colitis.

Defenders of the additive say that only "degraded" or non-food grade Carrageenan causes these effects and that the small amounts in food aren't harmful. Dr. Joanne Tobacman, physician-scientist at the University of Illinois College of Medicine, disagrees. Tobacman has been studying this controversial additive for over twenty years. In an address to a meeting of the National Organic Standards Board in April 2012, she testified that both undegraded and degraded carrageenan cause inflammation and that the amounts consumed in the human diets are sufficient to cause it.[30]

The Cornucopia Institute urges anyone suffering from gastrointestinal symptoms (Irritable Bowel syndrome/IBS, spastic colon, inflammatory bowel disease, chronic diarrhea, etc.) to completely eliminate carrageenan from the diet for two weeks.

The jury may still be out on this versatile additive, but one thing is almost certain. Increased scrutiny and tightening regulations on carrageenan have driven up prices in the food additive market, leading manufacturers to look for less expensive solutions. We'll probably be seeing less seaweed in our ice cream and more wood pulp.

Diacetyl

Diacetyl may not be special in being only one of the thousands of direct additives that appear in processed foods, but it's unique in another way. In having its own disease named after it. The lung condition, *Diacetyl Induced Bronchiolitis Obliterans*, is called "Popcorn Worker's Lung" due to the large number of microwave popcorn factory workers who have developed the respiratory illness. Since 2004, millions in damages have been awarded to popcorn workers who became sick from inhaling diacetyl fumes, but the disease can occur in any industry working with the chemical. In September 2012 the first consumer lawsuit surrounding diacetyl awarded 7.2 million in damages to Colorado resident Wayne Watson, who had eaten two bags of microwave popcorn daily over a period of 10 years.

The FDA still considers it a GRAS additive, but the National Institute for Occupational Safety and Health (OSHA) has suggested that diacetyl, when used in artificial butter flavoring (as used in many consumer foods), may be hazardous when heated and inhaled over a long period. The CDC has issued a safety alert for workers in factories that use diacetyl, and notes that toxicology studies have shown that vapors from heated butter flavorings can cause damage to airways in animals. California has legislation pending to ban diacetyl outright.

The European Union is taking a "wait and see approach" to the problem, pending further research, but U.S. companies are starting to voluntarily replace this ingredient in microwave popcorn. Major US manufacturers, like ConAgra and Pop Weaver, have stopped using the chemical in popcorn products.

Diacetyl does have some benefits. There's evidence that it works great as a mosquito repellant. Fruit flies avoid it, too.

Disodium Guanylate

A flavor enhancer commercially prepared from yeast extract, sea weed or sardines, disodium guanylate is often used in conjunction with MSG and added to instant noodles, potato chips and other snacks, savory rice, tinned vegetables, cured meats, and packaged soup. If a food contains disodium guanylate, it will likely contain MSG in some amount, even if monosodium glutamate is not listed on the label. Disodium guanylate is not safe for children under twelve weeks, and should generally be avoided by asthmatics and people with gout.

Monosodium Glutamate (MSG)

The most widely used flavor enhancer in the world, and easily the most controversial taste additive, is monosodium glutamate. Grandfathered in under the FDA's Group II, GRAS regulation, MSG has been under suspicion since 1968 when a letter published in *The New England Journal of Medicine* anecdotally described chest tightness and headache as a response to eating Chinese food. The letter's author, Dr. Robert Ho Man Kwok, labeled the cluster of symptoms "Chinese Restaurant Syndrome."

Similar complaints flooded the Food and Drug Administration and led to investigations into the safety of MSG, but several extensive reviews since 1970 have re-affirmed the safety of normal dosages of MSG, even for children. Despite the widespread belief that MSG can elicit a headache, nausea, and asthma-like symptoms, the association has never been demonstrated under rigorously controlled conditions. A 2006 review of 40 years' worth of literature on the subject found no clinical data to support the claim that MSG causes these symptoms.[31]

More recently, however, MSG has been implicated in the obesity epidemic. [32] [33] One obvious theory proposes that because MSG makes food taste better, people simply eat more when it's present. But in some studies the link between high MSG intake and being overweight holds even after accounting for the total number of calories people ate. There's some evidence to suggest that MSG might interfere with appetite-regulating systems in the body. [34] One study even speculates that this interference may begin even before birth if the mother is consuming processed foods that contain MSG. [35]

MSG in Disguise

As MSG has acquired increasingly bad publicity, manufacturers have turned to other flavor-enhancing additives which don't look as bad on the label but still contain free glutamic acid, just like MSG. A list of common MSG substitutes and of foods that most frequently contain MSG can be found in the Appendix.

Placing "No MSG," "No MSG Added," or "No Added MSG" on food labels has been deemed by the FDA to be false and misleading when the label also lists any hydrolyzed protein as an ingredient since it contains MSG. Thus, to advertise "No MSG," "No MSG Added," or "No Added MSG" when there is processed free glutamic acid (MSG) in a product is illegal. Given the over-burdened resources of the FDA, however, and the fact that new ingredients that contain MSG are invented and renamed every day, label violations are common.

Potassium Bromate

Potassium bromate is a flour conditioner used to strengthen dough and enable higher rising in bread baking. Under proper baking conditions, potassium bromate levels should be very low in finished bread products, but if too much is added, or if the product is not baked long enough or at adequate temperatures, more residual additive can remain. Foods containing high levels of potassium bromate can cause acute irritation to the gastrointestinal tract, resulting in nausea, vomiting, abdominal pain, and diarrhea. Outbreaks of gastrointestinal distress among schoolchildren have occurred after consumption of tortillas or burritos—breads which are usually baked for a shorter period of time and at lower temperatures than other bakery products.[36]

A powerful oxidizer, bromate was first found to cause tumors in rats in 1982.[37] Three decades of subsequent studies on rats and mice have confirmed that it causes tumors of the kidney, thyroid, and other organs. It is categorized as 2B (possibly carcinogenic to humans) by the International Agency for Research on Cancer and The World Health Organization has recommended its removal from all foods.

Although potassium bromate has been banned in many countries, the FDA has merely urged US manufacturers to voluntarily stop using it. Some manufacturers have moved to bromate-free processes, but the additive is still widely used in commercial bread products and by fast food chains.

The Center for Science in the Public Interest advises consumers to avoid bread, rolls, doughnuts, and cakes that list "potassium bromate" or "bromated flour" among their ingredients.

Propyl Gallate

Propyl gallate is another preservative used to slow the spoilage of fats and oils. It can be found in a host of foods including baked goods, shortening and vegetable oils, meat products, soup bases, mayonnaise and dried milk, candy and chewing gum. Propyl gallate has some antioxidant properties and laboratory studies have linked it to reductions in cancer, birth defects and dental cavities, but it is often used in conjunction with BHA and BHT because of the synergistic effects these preservatives have. It is another estrogen-mimicking compound.

Sulfites

Sulfites are preservatives commonly found in dried fruits and wines. For some consumers sulfites can cause allergic reactions like respiratory difficulty, headache, nausea, and digestive complaints. The FDA estimates that about one out of every 100 people is sensitive to the compounds. In 1986, the FDA banned the use of sulfites on whole foods and on fruits and vegetables that are eaten raw, but allowed them in processed foods, assuming that manufacturers reveal their presence on product labels. Sulfites may appear on ingredients lists as sulfur dioxide, potassium bisulfite, potassium metabisulfite, or sodium sulfite.

Food Color Additives

The practice of coloring foods has existed for thousands of years. Spices like paprika, saffron and turmeric were used to color food 3,000 years ago and vegetables, flowers, even ores and minerals, have been used to color foods throughout recorded history. Today we enjoy dying Easter Eggs and decorating our birthday cakes and holiday cookies with brightly colored frostings. In theory, food colorings are fun. They allow us to express our creativity and to make food presentations more interesting. What's not so fun is the extent to which synthetic colors are added to modern processed foods. The FDA says that Americans consume five times as much food dye as we did thirty years ago. These colors are added to our food for an array of purposes, but almost none of them have anything to do with nutrition.

Most of us realize, if we're made to think about it, that the riot of colors that fills a package of M&Ms or a box of Fruit Loops is the result of artificial food colorings (AFCs). Far fewer of us are aware that many seemingly "natural" foods such as oranges and salmon are sometimes also dyed to mask natural variations in color. As a Floridian myself, I was particularly distressed to learn that our state's fabled citrus crop is routinely injected with Citrus Red 2, a dye used to make the oranges a brighter and more uniform color. Citrus Red 2 is banned in most of the world because it is a known carcinogen. It is not even approved by our own FDA for actual ingestion. The FDA allows its use in oranges, justifying that the dye never permeates the peel into the pulp or fruit. Obviously, the FDA doesn't expect us to cook with whole oranges or segments or to zest the peel.

Artificial food colorings are often used in this way, to intensify natural colors and make them more appealing. That neon red maraschino cherry atop your chocolate cake or floating in your cocktail? Without Red Dye No. 4, it would be a much less appetizing grayish beige. The color, by the way, was banned in 1960, along with Red Number 1 and Yellow Numbers 1 through 4. It was restored five years later when such cherries were determined to be for decoration, not eating.

Color is an integral part of the multi-sensory experience that makes up taste for humans and in some instances is the strongest identifier of a food. It's an association that manufacturers know how to exploit. The chemical coloring box, good for making red cherries redder and oranges more orange, is increasingly used to mask or conceal the fact that the associative food doesn't even exist in the modern product we're purchasing. Breakfast cereals, bagels, toaster pastries, muffin mixes and other products frequently contain small bits made of artificial colors, hydrogenated oils, and liquid sugars that may *look* like fruit, but aren't at all. Kellogg's, General Mills, and Betty Crocker are among the companies that fake blueberries and strawberries with petro-chemical dyes.

Color Additive Health Risks

The practice of using artificial colorings to fake fruit is deceitful. But to some consumers these colorings may also be dangerous. Food colorings have been linked to hyperactivity in children for more than fifty years. In some people the dyes can trigger allergic reactions or compound the problems of aspirin sensitivity. According to The Center for Science in the Public Interest, food dyes pose a rainbow of risks.

Hyperactivity

A link between food dyes and hyperactivity in children was first suggested in 1973 when Dr. Benjamin Feingold presented research to the AMA implicating food additives in learning and behavior disorders.[38] His research, based on over 1,200 cases and including over 3,000 different food additives, led to the development of a food elimination program known as The Feingold Diet. [39]

Feingold's work has been ridiculed and some subsequent studies did appear to disprove his position. Others, however, have supported his hypothesis. Many medical professionals and parents remain convinced that the Feingold Diet leads to significant decreases in symptoms of hyperactivity.

In September 2007, a study published by the prestigious British journal *The Lancet* found evidence to suggest that a mix of artificial food colors and additives may exacerbate hyperactivity in children. [29] In the following year The Center for Science in the Public Interest, with support of a long list of scientists and researchers, petitioned the FDA to revoke its approval for blue, green, orange, red and yellow dyes linked to behavioral changes in hyperactive children.

In 2011 the FDA responded by convening an advisory committee to discuss the risks. Despite the testimony of parents who described significant improvement in their children's behavior after withdrawal of AFCs, the committee decided that there was insufficient evidence to support a link between artificial dyes in foods and children with ADHD. The committee made no recommendations for banning or regulating dye additives found in food products, but acknowledged the trend with artificial dyes and side effects in children and suggested that more research is needed.

A research review published in *The Journal of Child and Adolescent Health* found evidence for the fact that the removal of artificial dyes had substantial positive effects on the behavior of children with ADHD as well as on children from the general population without ADHD. [40]

Allergic Reactions

Some food dyes have been implicated in allergic reactions and in triggering asthma episodes. Yellow dye #5 (Tartrazine) appears to cause the most allergic and intolerance reactions of all the azo dyes, particularly among asthmatics and those with an aspirin intolerance. Brilliant Blue #2 has also been linked to allergic responses.

Identifying Color Additives

There are currently nine certified color additives approved for food use in the United States; seven for general use in food, two for exteriors of food. Each color tends to be derived from several ingredients, and comes in generally two forms.

Dye form tends to produce less vibrant colors, is more likely to bleed, and is not soluble in oil. This form is used in beverages, dry mixes, baked goods, confections, dairy products, pet foods and a variety of other products.

Lake form is oil soluble, tends to be more stable and does not bleed. Lakes forms are used in coated tablets, cookie fillings, candies, and other products in which color bleeding would be undesirable. They will be listed on an ingredient label with FD&C, for Food, Drug and Cosmetic, preceding the color.

Example: *FD&C Blue #1.*

They may also appear abbreviated, with just the color, Blue 1, or with "Lake" following the color name.

Example: *Blue 1 Lake.*

The European Union uses E numbers as codes for chemicals which can be used as food additives for use within the European Union.

Example: *E133 Brilliant Blue FCF*

It's important for parents to be able to identify color additives in foods. In the Appendix of this book you'll find a detailed **Colorings and Dyes Chart** listing the common uses of these chemicals and their known health risks.

Insect-based Colors

Not every color additive is purely synthetic. Spices, vegetable juice, fruits, seeds, or caramelized sugar may be used to heighten or change the color appearance of processed foods, but some of the "natural" sources for color alteration are also suspect. Two forms of coloring, cochineal extract and carmine, are derived from female cochineal beetles, which are raised in primarily in Peru and the Canary Islands. These insects provide a pink, red, or purple color to foods ranging from ice cream and yogurt to fruit drinks and are also used in pharmaceuticals and cosmetics.

Food colorings made from bugs are problematic for vegetarians as well as for people whose religious or dietary laws preclude eating animals, but they are also a concern for that subset of the population for whom they have the potential to provoke severe allergic reactions. Currently, they may be declared on labels as "artificial color" or "color added." Labels declaring "color produced from insects" are not likely to catch on.

Progress on Color Additives

The color front is one place in the Great American Food Fight where we're scoring some victories. Companies like Pepperidge Farm have reformulated their "Goldfish Colors" and "Goldfish Colors Neon" snacks, to replace the red and blue dyes that had colored these products with beet, watermelon, turmeric and paprika extracts. In January 2011, Frito-lay upped the ante, announcing that half of their products would be "all natural." Frito-lay now offers Sun Chips colored with Paprika and their White Cheddar Cheetoes no longer feature neon orange stain. New England-based Necco Wafers is also onboard, now producing candies colored with purple cabbage, red beets and cocoa powder. A consumer campaign recently convinced Starbucks to stop using cochineal extract to color its strawberry-flavored drinks.

These are great examples of consumer power at work. With continuing pressure, and more grocery story ballots that refuse to vote for unnecessary and possibly toxic color additives, there may come a day when this issue will be history.

In the appendix of this book, you will find a chart that lists the commonly used food colorings and known associations with disease or health risks. Links to printable copies of this and other charts can be found at the www.GreatAmericanFoodFight.com website.

Eating in the Meantime

- Any prepared food including a powder packet or a sauce will almost certainly contain MSG. Almost all prepared soups contain MSG.

- If you write or call a manufacturer about this issue, ask for specific information about "free glutamic acid." Don't settle for just being told "no MSG," or that the additive is "natural."

- There's certainly no need to forego the frosted birthday cake or the colorful Christmas cookies. The takeaway information for parents is that color additives don't have to be a routine addition to daily meals.

- The experiences of family visits to orchards, gardens, or organic farms can go a long way toward raising consciousness to the fact that fruits and vegetables, like people, can still be wonderful without necessarily looking "perfect."

- If your child suffers from asthma or other respiratory conditions, has an aspirin sensitivity, or has been diagnosed with hyperactivity disorder, why take the risk? Until further research assures us of their safety, artificial dyes and colors are among the easiest additives to eliminate.

- Work to overcome your own resistance, and to teach your children, that whole, organic foods are not always the perfect cartoon images depicted on Saturday morning TV and the front of label packaging. Whole foods have imperfections and natural color variations. Color is not necessarily an indicator of ripeness or quality or taste.

- Experiment with using natural food colorings from your own pantry or fridge. Beet juice, coffee, cocoa powder, purple carrots or cabbage, avocado, saffron, turmeric and thawed frozen berries can tint icings.

- Organic produce will not contain food dyes. Nor will whole-grain flour or unsweetened natural dairy products.

- Remember that colorings are used almost solely in foods of low nutritional value. There's very little to lose by avoiding them as much as possible.

- Support those retailers like Trader Joes and Whole Foods who refuse to carry petroleum-based dyes such as Red 40, Blue 1 and Yellow 5 and 6, and those manufacturers who are making the move to more natural colorings in their products.

- Anyone suffering from gastrointestinal symptoms (irritable bowel syndrome/IBS, spastic colon, inflammatory bowel disease, chronic diarrhea, etc.) should consider eliminating carrageenan from the diet to determine if it might be a factor in causing the symptoms.

- Check the ingredients list on bread products. It's becoming easier to find bakers who forego potassium bromate.

Chapter 5. The Big Fat Lies about Fat

Some diet myths can be really stubborn. That one about nighttime calories being somehow more caloric than day calories is an especially persistent one. The notion that certain foods, like grapefruit, can actually "burn" calories is another. But the fallacies surrounding fat are downright tenacious. Eradicating the myth that fat, especially saturated fat, is bad for us is going to take some doing. It's a myth, after all, that's been perpetuated for at least the last half-century with the enthusiastic support of the media, the medical and academic communities, nutritionists and health organizations, our own government, and, of course, the food manufacturers who've profited mightily from keeping it alive.

But the fight to finally vanquish this stubborn myth, and to correct the widespread misinformation about fats in general, is well worth the struggle. For many, the knowledge that eating fat doesn't cause heart disease, that it doesn't cause cancer, indeed, the knowledge that eating fat *doesn't even make you fat*, will come as shocking, as well as guilt-relieving, news. For some, it just might be life-saving information.

To understand how the fat myths became so entrenched, we need to go back more than half a century. We need to return to the post war years and to the work of one particular researcher. In reviewing the origins of the big fat lies about fat we'll also, not coincidentally, be reviewing the history of the obesity epidemic, too.

The Big Fat Lie about Heart Disease

The years after World War II had seen a precipitous rise in the incidence of myocardial infarction (heart attack) among American business executives. The lifestyles of these big city businessmen were sedentary, and stressful, and they were smoking like crazy (think *Mad Men*), but for many doctors and scientists the most likely culprit for all those clogged arteries had to be diet.

One idea—that saturated fat and cholesterol in the blood was the cause of heart disease—had been proposed as far back as the mid nineteenth century. For American nutritionist Ancel Keys, this was the diet/heart theory that made the most sense and he set out to prove it. Keys studied the dietary patterns of seven countries, subsequently publishing, in 1953, a paper proposing that saturated fats and cholesterol in the blood were the major contributors to heart disease deaths.

Key's theory, now known as the Lipid Hypothesis, was received in a flood of rave reviews. Most everyone ignored the fact that no primary research had been undertaken to support the thesis as well as the massive inconsistencies and contradictions in the data. The study's biggest flaw, however, was the data that wasn't there. In the seven countries which Keys studied, a higher saturated fat intake did, indeed, equate to higher rates of heart disease. But Keys completely ignored the data from 15 other countries which had high intakes of saturated fat but *low* incidence of cardiovascular disease. That data would have seriously undermined his theory, but it might have saved countless lives.

In a very few years Keys' diet/heart theory became the accepted gospel in the nutrition community. The American Medical Association, the American Heart Association, public health officials, and eventually Congress, swallowed the Lipid Hypothesis hook, line and sinker. In 1970, a congressional committee led by Senator George McGovern issued a groundbreaking report advising Americans to lower their risk of heart disease by eating less fat.

With "fat" identified as Public Enemy Number 1 in the American diet, food manufacturers got busy. The race was on to produce low-fat and no-fat foods, and to chemically engineer the saturated fat out of just about everything. During the decade of the 90s, the food industry introduced more than 1,000 reduced-fat food products each year, many of which bore little resemblance, physically or nutritionally, to the whole foods our grandparents knew. Consumers were really worried about fat, and the processed food industry was eager to calm those worries.

> By the mid-70s the low fat revolution had been well launched. Unfortunately, so had the obesity epidemic

There was one obstacle, however. Fat really tastes good! If that tasty fat came out, something else would have to replace it. Hydrogenated oils were one option. Sugar was another. With the invention of high-fructose corn syrup, adding that sweetness was now really easy, and really cheap. Both substitutes found their way into thousands of foods, along with a pinch, sometimes much more than a pinch, of salt. The new way of eating caught on. Americans were advised to cut back on animal fat, butter, and tropical oils. Lots of "fast" carbohydrates made from sugar, refined grains, or starch took their place.

But how did that advice work out? Let's look at a very simple comparison chart that illustrates the changes over five decades:

	1960	2010
Percent of calories from fats and oils	45%	33%
Percent of population obese	13%	34%
Percent of population with Type 2 diabetes	<1%	8%

Clearly, there was something wrong with the notion that simply reducing our fat intake would make us healthier. The growing number of fat-modified products on the market paralleled the rising obesity rates. Americans weren't getting thinner, and they were far less healthy.

The Big Fat House of Cards

Association never proves causation. The proposition that saturated fats *per se* cause heart disease was not just too easy, but for many experts, it was just plain wrong. There was Dr. Weston Price, a dentist whose global travels and research into pre-industrial populations had convinced him that diet was the main source, not just of tooth decay, but of most Western diseases.[41] His book, *Nutritional and Physical Deterioration*, inspired Sally Fallon to found the Weston Price Foundation in 1999. This non-profit is still dedicated to restoring nutrient-dense foods to the human diet. It was co-founded by Dr. Mary G. Enig, an internationally recognized expert in lipid biochemistry, who has spent a lifetime challenging government assertions that dietary animal fat causes cancer and heart disease.[42]

Danish researcher Uffe Ravnskov is another skeptic who has battled the lipid hypothesis throughout his medical and academic career. Since 1990, Ravnskov has published over 80 scientific papers critical of the hypotheses.[43] He contends that "the successful dissemination of the diet-heart idea is due to authors systematically ignoring or misquoting discordant (contradictory) studies"[44]

There are many, many others—from cardiologists and neuroscientists, to popular food experts like Michael Pollan, who don't agree that that the consumption of fat and dietary cholesterol lead to a higher rate of coronary disease.[45, 46] Research that challenges the lipid hypothesis is abundant, but you will rarely hear it mentioned.

In 2007, Marion Volk undertook a comprehensive examination of Key's study and the subsequent studies that are still held out as proof of the validity of the lipid hypothesis. She observes that the association between saturated fat consumption and heart disease has been repeated so often that it has gained the status of fact. She notes that the constant citation of certain studies introduces bias into subsequent ones.[47]

The most frequently cited of those studies, The Framingham Heart Study, began in 1948 and followed 6,000 people at five-year intervals. While many insights, including knowledge about lifestyle habits and the psychosocial factors that contribute to heart disease, have come out of this study, the Framingham Study did not, as so many still assume, support the lipid hypothesis.

In a 1992 article published in the *Archives of Internal Medicine*, William Castelli, the study's director, admitted that results were unexpected. "In Framingham, Mass," wrote Castelli, ". . . we found that the people who ate the most cholesterol, ate the most saturated fat, ate the most calories, weighed the least and were the most physically active." [48]

Indeed, the Framingham study found nothing that the researchers expected. The study revealed no association between percent of calories from fat and serum cholesterol levels and no indication of a relationship between dietary cholesterol and serum cholesterol level. There was, in short, no suggestion of any relationship between diet and the subsequent development of heart disease in the study group.[49] Yet, this is the bedrock science on which the entire "fat will kill you" conventional wisdom came to rest. It is still the basis for the nearly ubiquitous health advice to avoid saturated fats.

In the intervening years since Framingham, more research has exonerated the role of saturated fat in the development of heart disease. In a 1996 cohort follow-up study of more than 43,000 health professionals from 1986 until 1994, researchers concluded that the data gleaned from the study "do not support the strong association between intake of saturated fat and risk of coronary heart disease"[50] The National Institute of Health spent several hundred million dollars trying to demonstrate a connection between fat consumption and heart disease, but five major studies revealed no such a link. A sixth, however, costing well over $100 million alone, concluded that reducing cholesterol by drug therapy could prevent heart disease.[45]

Results of The Women's Health Initiative Dietary Modification Trial, which included almost 49,000 women, were published in *The Journal of the American Medical Association* in 2006. The study found virtually identical rates of heart attack, stroke, and other forms of cardiovascular disease in women who followed a low-fat diet and in those women who didn't. And women on the low-fat diet didn't lose, or gain, any more weight than women who followed their usual diets.[51]

In a very recent meta-analysis researchers collected data from 21 independent studies that included almost 350,000 people, about 11,000 of whom developed cardiovascular disease. The study, published in the *American Journal of Clinical Nutrition* in January, 2010, found **"no relationship between the intake of saturated fat and the incidence of heart disease or stroke."** (Emphasis mine.) In fact, the "risk ratio" for the development of CVD as intake of saturated fat increased was 1.0, indicating that people who ate more saturated fat were no more or less likely to develop CVD.[52]

Overall, the data from clinical trials and epidemiology simply do not support an independent role for saturated fat in the determination of CVD risk.

Far too many average Americans, however, aren't getting this message. We still don't understand why the "fat-free" foods that we consume don't help us lose weight. We're still fat-phobic and we're still paying the price. The low fat revolution has given an entire generation of Americans a nutritional myopia that still hasn't been corrected. The demonization of fat continues, to the benefit of Big Food and Big Pharma, but to the detriment of public health.

The Role of Fat

Fat is the most concentrated of the three nutrients that create fuel for our bodies. Fats provide 9 calories per gram, more than twice the number provided by carbohydrates or protein. They are important for insulating the body, for controlling inflammation, for blood clotting, and brain development. Healthy skin and hair are maintained by fat. Fat helps the body absorb and move the vitamins A, D, E, and K through the bloodstream. They lubricate our joints, regulate our hormones, and provide the essential fatty acids (EFAs), linoleic and linolenic acid, which cannot be made by the body and must be obtained from food. Quite simply we can't live without fat. But all fats aren't created equal.

Types of Fat

All fatty acids are carbon atom chains with hydrogen atoms attached to the carbon atoms. There are three main types of fatty acids: saturated, monounsaturated, and polyunsaturated.

Saturated Fats

Saturated fats are so-called because, chemically speaking, their carbon atoms are "saturated" with the most hydrogen atoms possible on the long carbon chain. Because this chemical structure results in no empty spaces, the molecules of saturated fats are packed tightly together and tend to be solid or semi-solid at room temperature. These are very stable molecules and resist oxidation. Normally they do not turn rancid, even when heated. Saturated fats are mainly found in animal products like meat, dairy, eggs and seafood, but some plant foods are also high in saturated fats.

For at least the last fifty years, as health authorities cautioned about the consumption of saturated fats, some of these, like coconut oil, for example, which can be as high as 92% saturated, have been given particularly bad press. Unfortunately, however, the American public has been fed a great deal of misinformation on saturated fats and that disservice has shown up in exactly what the experts hoped to avoid—a far greater incidence of coronary heart disease and exploding obesity rates. Natural saturated fats are not unhealthy. The only saturated fat that is even remotely dangerous is oxidized fat damaged as a result of high heat, lengthy air exposure, or food processing.

But it *is* true that some fats are bad for us. In order to understand which ones, we must know something about the chemistry of fat and the ways they work together.

Monounsaturated Fats

From a chemical standpoint, monounsaturated fats (MUFAs) are simply fats that have one double-bonded (unsaturated) carbon in the molecule. Typically these fats are liquid at room temperature, but become solid when chilled. Monounsaturated fats come mainly from plant sources. Avocados and olives are rich sources of monounsaturated fats, as are nuts (hazelnuts, macadamia nuts, pecans, almonds, pistachios and cashews) and many plant seeds (sesame, sunflower, pumpkin and flax.). Some legumes, but especially peanuts, are high in MUFA content. Most fish, but especially Atlantic pickled herring, halibut, sablefish, and mackerel, are rich food sources of monounsaturated fats. Butter, eggs and many varieties of cheese are also good food sources.

Polyunsaturated Fats

Unlike the other types of fat, polyunsaturated fats (PUFAs) are chemically linked by multiple double bonds. Because of the bends and turns at the site of these bonds, PUFAs don't bind readily, a quality that keeps them liquid, even inside the refrigerator, but also makes them highly unstable and vulnerable to oxidation. During processing, and when exposed to heat and light, detached molecules, or "free radicals," react quickly with other compounds, trying to capture the needed electron to gain stability. Generally, these free radicals attack the nearest stable molecule, "stealing" its electron, but thereby creating a new free radical in a chain reaction that, once started, can eventually result in the disruption of living cells. Free radical production causes the inflammation that has been linked to cancer and other degenerative diseases and may even be the source of aging itself. Unfortunately, most of the fats in the Western diet are now derived from polyunsaturated oils made from soy, corn, safflower and canola.

Polyunsaturates are further divided in Omega 6 and Omega-3 polyunsaturates, and here it's all about the balance.

Essential Fatty Acids: Omegas 3, 6, and 9

Of the Omega polyunsaturates, two are considered critical, or essential, for human nutrition. Omega-3 fatty acids (also called w-3, or n-3) and Omega-6 fatty acids (also called w-6, or n-6) are considered essential because humans cannot synthesize them from scratch. We must obtain them from our diets.

While the human genetic code has remained the same for millennia, our diets have changed radically and rapidly. We evolved on diets very high in Omega-3 fats from the green plants, fruits, nuts, berries, fish and lean meat that our Paleolithic ancestors consumed. By contrast, our diets today are high in the intake of Omega-6 fats, obtained from cereals and processed and refined oils.

Anthropological and epidemiological evidence shows that humans evolved on a diet with a ratio of Omega-6 to Omega-3 essential fatty acids as close as one to one. (The dietary ratio of Omega-6 to Omega-3 fatty acids was one to two only about 60 years ago.) Today, however, the typical North American diet may contain 11 to 30 times more Omega-6 fatty acids than mega-3 fatty acids.

This escalating imbalance is important in the development of what may be called, without irony, the "diseases of civilization." Excessive amounts of Omega-6 PUFAs promote the pathogenesis of many diseases, including cardiovascular disease, cancer, arthritis, and autoimmune diseases, all of which are believed to stem from inflammation in the body.[i] Mounting evidence also links these fatty acids to psychological disorders, including depression, hyperactivity, and even a tendency toward violence.[ii] Increased levels of Omega-3 PUFAs, on the other hand, exert suppressive, or braking, effects on these diseases and conditions.

Two of the Omega-3s seem to be especially important for the protection they offer against disease. **DHA** (docosahexaenoic acid) and **EPA** (eicosapentaenoic acid) help reduce the risk of heart attacks, lower blood triglyceride levels, help to prevent stroke and are critical in visual and neurological development. DHA, the major Omega-3 fatty acid in the brain, appears to be protective against Alzheimer's disease. They're found most abundantly in fatty fish like salmon and sardines.

The third Omega-3 fat, **ALA** (alinolenic acid), doesn't protect the heart as much as DHA and EPA does. Most Americans get enough ALA from margarine, salad dressing, and other foods made with vegetable oils.

More evidence is needed on the ideal ratio of Omega-3 to Omega-6 polyunsaturates. But a large body of scientific research suggests that increasing the Omega-3 fatty acids may have a number of health benefits.

Trans Fats and Hydrogenation

We come now to a discussion of a type of fat that we can unequivocally say is "bad" for you. Trans fats (TFAs) are manufactured through a process called hydrogenation, whereby hydrogen molecules are forced into oil molecules through the use of intense heat, high pressure and toxic catalysts like nickel. The result is a fat more solid than oil, making it less likely to spoil and thus giving a longer shelf life to processed and manufactured foods.

Manufactured Trans fats were first introduced to the American public during World War II when butter was rationed, and gained widespread acceptance in the 50s and 60s. The Low Fat Revolution of the next decades spurred manufacturers to substitute Trans fats and partially hydrogenated Trans fats for natural solid fats in the fast food, snack food, bakery and processed food industries.

By the 90s, however, research began to expose Trans fats as culpable in many diseases, including CVD, diabetes, and cancers. Even obesity was linked to the consumption of Trans fats rather than the much aligned saturated fats.

In March 2003, Denmark became the first country in the world to ban all but very small quantities of Trans fat in food. Heart disease rates in Denmark have subsequently declined by more than 20%.[53] Trans fat labeling on food packaging became mandatory in the US in 2008 and some US states have enacted their own bans.

Following a lawsuit and a considerable amount of public pressure the FDA promised, in 2013, to ban Trans fats but as of this writing the proposed rule still has not been finalized.

The good fats vs. bad fats debate has been grossly over-simplified and is erroneously presented so that saturated fats and Trans fats are conflated and grouped together as the "bad" fats. The truth is that natural, undamaged fats are absolutely necessary for human health and development, whereas there is no safe level of Trans fats.

Solid Cooking Fats

Solid fats come naturally only from animal foods, but vegetable oils can be made solid through the hydrogenation process. Beef and poultry fat are still used for cooking, but the most commonly used solid fats are lard, shortening, butter, and margarine.

Lard

Your grandma probably cooked with lard, the rendered pork fat still used for cooking in many traditional cultures. It's making something of an American comeback now that more scientists and consumers are becoming enlightened about the dangers of Trans fats. Lard's high smoke point, 400°F/200°C, makes it suitable for deep frying. It gives a light airiness to baked goods that is hard to duplicate.

Shortening

The first hydrogenated imitation food to be introduced to the American public was Crisco, developed by Proctor and Gamble as a means to maximize cottonseed profits. By adding hydrogen atoms to the fatty acid chain, chemists found that hardened oil could be used to make candles and soap, but by happy coincidence, at least for Proctor and Gamble, the solid product had the appearance and properties of lard. There was even more profit potential in selling it as food.

A masterful and highly effective marketing campaign, and a free cookbook, soon convinced consumers that Crisco was a healthier alternative to cooking with animal fats and more economical to use than butter. Crisco quickly supplanted lard in the nation's kitchens, and Trans fat shortenings entered the manufacturing process of millions of foods.

In 2007 all Crisco products were reformulated to contain less than one gram of Trans fat per serving, The all-vegetable shortening contains soybean oil, fully hydrogenated palm oil, partially hydrogenated palm and soybean oils, and stabilizers. There are many other similar "no Trans fats" shortenings now on the market.

Consumers should be aware, however, that Trans fat levels of less than 0.5 grams per serving can still be listed as containing 0 grams Trans fat on the food label.

Butter

Real butter, of course, is a dairy product. A full discussion of cow's milk, from which most commercial butter is made, is taken up in Chapter 7, but any examination of solid fats must include butter, the cooking fat, spread, and condiment of choice of many cultures for millennia.

Because butter has more cholesterol than other fats, it has suffered more than any other traditional food from the big fat lies about fats. It is not, however, the artery clogger that it's reputed to be. In fact, the history of butter consumption runs completely counter to the obesity epidemic.

> Because butter has more has more cholesterol than other fats, it has suffered more than any other traditional food from the big fat lies about fats.

In the US and the United Kingdom butter was actually rationed during and immediately after World War II—that precise time period when ischemic heart conditions reached alarming proportions. By mid-century, however, margarine had overtaken butter, and, by 2000, we were consuming three times more margarine than butter.

The good news is that butter sales are now reviving as consumers learn that those highly processed hydrogenated spreads and oils were a move in the wrong direction.

Commercial butter is 80–82% milk fat, 16–17% water, and 1–2 percent milk solids, or curd. Reduced-fat, or "light," butter usually contains about 40 percent milk fat. Butter has a good balance of Omega-3s to Omega-6s and also contains protein, calcium, phosphorous (about 1.2%) and fat-soluble vitamins A, D and E.

Margarine

Margarine is manufactured by forcing pressurized hydrogen gas into vegetable oil, usually soy or corn, with the aid of a heavy metal catalyst. At the end of the hydrogenation process, the margarine must be bleached, deodorized, artificially flavored, and dyed yellow to approximate the appearance of real butter. The resulting spread is a highly artificial fat, now containing dangerous Trans fatty acids, but missing the essential fatty acids, with about the same calorie count as butter.

For fifty years American consumers have been urged to substitute margarine for butter to reduce the risk of heart disease. But heart disease is still our number one killer, and recently analyzed data from 1966 to 1973 indicates that replacing butter and other saturated fats with vegetable oils may have increased the risk of heart disease instead of reducing it. The National Institute of Health analysis studied data on 458 men who had cardiovascular disease. Those who had dietary advice and replaced saturated fats in their diets with polyunsaturated vegetable oils had a 16 percent rate of dying from heart disease compared to a 10 percent death rate for those men who weren't told to change their diets.[54]

Many table spreads today are made from blends of margarine and butter. Some experts have likened switching to soft margarines to smoking a low tar cigarette.

Cooking Oils

The almost bewildering proliferation of cooking oils is certainly part of the low fat revolution. Supermarkets now carry dozens of types and varieties and many more boutique oils are available at health food stores and specialty grocers.

What follows are some of the most commonly used oils that are now substituted for lard or butter on the table, and in baking, frying and sautéing. You should be aware that heat will destroy many of the health benefits of these oils. You should also keep in mind that most generic vegetable oils and margarines used in restaurants and in processed foods in North America are made from soy, corn, canola, or cottonseed. Unless these oils specifically say "Non-GMO" or "Organic," they are probably genetically modified. See Chapter 8 for a discussion on genetically modified crop plants. Finally, readers should note that the fatty acid compositions of these oils can vary, depending on the source of the oils

Avocado Oil

(12% Saturated; 70 % Monounsaturated, 70% Polyunsaturated)

One of the few edible oils not derived from seeds, avocado oil is pressed from the fleshy pulp surrounding the avocado pit. It has an extremely high smoke point (520°F), especially when refined. Avocado oil has a healthy, monounsaturated fat content (71%) and is rich in vitamins B, C and E, as well as several minerals. Ounce for ounce, avocados contain 60% more potassium than bananas. Avocado oil has a mild flavor and works well as a carrier for other flavors.

Canola Oil

(7.4% Saturated; 63.3% Monounsaturated, 28.1% Polyunsaturated)

Canola is new to the oil market. So new, in fact, that it dates only to about 1978, when the Canadian oil industry genetically modified the rapeseed plant to produce oil for human consumption. The new crop was named Canola, an acronym made from Canada oil, low acid. By

1985 it had been given GRAS status by the FDA—a feat rumored to have cost the Canadian government $50 million dollars, and canola soon became the Cinderella oil for fat-phobic consumers.

Reports on the dangers of canola oil are widespread on the internet. Some are based on the fact that rapeseed belongs to the brassica or mustard family. But this plant is not the source of the mustard gas used in chemical warfare. Reports of allergies and other reactions to canola oil have also surfaced on the internet, but none have been reported in medical journals. While you may read otherwise, canola was not the cause of the Mad Cow outbreak in Great Britain in the 90s.

A more legitimate concern is the fact that canola oil must be partially hydrogenated or refined before it is used commercially and thus can be a source of high levels of Trans fatty acids. While canola does have a favorable ratio of Omega-6 to Omega-3 (about 3:1), most of the Omega-3 in canola oil is transformed into Trans fat during the deodorization process.

A 1997 study found that that piglets fed milk replacement containing canola oil showed signs of vitamin E deficiency.[55] There is also some evidence that canola retards growth in laboratory animals, which is why the FDA does not allow canola in infant formula.

Coconut Oil

(86% Saturated; 6% Monounsaturated; 2% Polyunsaturated)

Of all the much-maligned saturated fats, coconut oil has been subject to the most negative, and error-filled, publicity. Back in the 1930s, Dr. Weston Price found South Pacific Islanders whose diets were high in coconut to be healthy and trim, despite high dietary fat, and heart disease was virtually non-existent. Fifty years later, researchers studying two Polynesian communities for whom coconut was the primary caloric energy source found them to have excellent cardiovascular health and fitness. (2)

Coconut oil is a significant source of lauric acid, the antimicrobial in human milk known to fights bacteria and viruses. Organic virgin coconut oil does not oxidize, even at high temperatures, and can keep up to two years. The partially hydrogenated varieties, however, will contain Trans fats.

Cottonseed Oil

(26% Saturated; 18% Monounsaturated; 52%, Polyunsaturated)

After soy, corn and canola, cotton is the fourth genetically modified crop for the extraction of oil. It is cheap to produce and has a long shelf life, making it an obvious choice for inclusion in processed foods. It is popularly used in mayonnaise and salad dressings, and raw as a salad oil. Cottonseed oil is high in vitamins E and K, but it is typically hydrogenated, which makes it mildly inflammatory, and there are other drawbacks to its consumption.

Cotton seeds contain natural toxins which protect the plants from insect infestation. One of these is the compound, gossypol, which for decades has been demonstrated to be detrimental to animal and human fertility. Gossypol is used as a male contraceptive in China, Africa and Brazil.[56] The finished oil is refined, bleached, and deodorized to reduce gossypol levels.

Finally, because cotton seeds are molecularly similar to peanuts, some people who are allergic to peanuts or gluten may have a reaction to cottonseed oil. No labeling of cottonseed oil as a potential allergen is required.

Corn Oil

(13% Saturated; 27% Monounsaturated; 54% Polyunsaturated)

Corn oil is extracted from the germ of the corn, or maize, plant. Cheap to produce, thanks to agricultural subsidies, it has a very high smoke point and resists rancidity. It is ubiquitous in processed foods, and the oil of choice for frying in the fast food industries. Corn oil contains a high amount of Omega-6 fatty acids. The majority of brands sold in the United States will be manufactured from genetically modified corn.

Flaxseed Oil

(9% Saturated; 20% Monounsaturated; 66% Polyunsaturated)

Flaxseed oil comes from the seeds of the flax, or linseed plant. Flaxseed oil contains the highest plant-based levels of the Omega-3 fatty acids, about 57%, so it's the best choice among the oils for getting some fat balance in your diet. It is a healthy finishing oil, and may be used in salad dressings, spreads or dips, or added to prepared foods, but it should not be used for frying or cooking. Flaxseed oil is easily destroyed by heat, light, and oxygen and turns rancid without refrigeration. Products that may contain flaxseed oil include cereal, bread and other baked goods.

Grape Seed Oil

(11% Saturated; 70% Polyunsaturated; 11%, Monounsaturated 16%)

As abundant byproducts of winemaking, grape seeds have been pressed for their oil for centuries. The high smoke point (485 F) makes it suitable for hot food preparation, and grape oil also has excellent emulsification properties, making it ideal for dressings that don't cloud or separate when chilled. Grape seed oils, however, are very high in in Omega-6 polyunsaturated fatty acids.

Olive Oil

(13% Saturated; 73% Monounsaturated; 10% Polyunsaturated)

Olive oil is among the healthiest of all the cooking oils, offering a good balance of both monounsaturated and polyunsaturated fats. Extra virgin olive oil, however, which is generally considered healthiest and best tasting, can have a very low smoke point, sometimes listed at only 220 Fahrenheit (105 Celsius), making it unsuitable for frying. Use regular olive oil for cooking, and extra virgin olive oil for salads and other uncooked foods.

Palm Oil

(49% Saturated; 37% Monounsaturated; 9% Polyunsaturated)

Palm oil is derived from the pulp of the oil palm fruit, whereas palm kernel oil is obtained from the pressing of the palm seed.

Opinions on the health benefits of palm oil are confusing and controversial with various papers arguing for, and against, the relative safety of palm oil as a replacement for Trans fats. It's clear that populations living in the tropical areas have enjoyed palm oil for centuries without suffering the detriments of heart disease to the extent they are today as they adopt the western diet and lifestyle.

Palm oil contains several disease-fighting antioxidants (tocotrienols, tocopherols, vitamin E and beta-carotene). It is stable and will not break down at high temperatures.

Ecology-minded consumers should know, however, that there are serious environmental concerns surrounding production of palm oil. Clearance for palm oil is a leading cause of deforestation and the destruction of orangutan habitat.

Peanut Oil

(16% Saturated; 46% Monounsaturated; 32% Polyunsaturated)

Like olive oil, peanut oil is relatively stable and has a high smoking point, making it appropriate for occasional stir-fry cooking. The high Omega-6 content of peanut oil, however, means that its use should be limited.

Unrefined, "gourmet," "aromatic," or cold pressed oils may still contain the proteins that cause reactions in individuals who are allergic to peanuts. Research shows, however, that highly refined peanut oil, which has had all of the allergic proteins removed, does not cause an allergic response. A controlled human study published in *The British Medical Journal* that tested refined peanut oil in 60 severely allergic individuals, found that "refined peanut oil did not pose a risk in any of the subjects" who were allergic to peanuts.

The FDA Food Allergen Labeling and Consumer Protection Act of 2004 and the Federal Food, Drug, and Cosmetic Act excludes highly refined oils and ingredients derived from highly refined oils from the definition of "major food allergen."

Safflower Oil

(8% Saturated; 13% Monounsaturated; 79% Polyunsaturated)

Made from the seeds of the safflower plant which grows mainly in arid areas of India, Iran, and North Africa, safflower oil has long been consumed for medicinal benefits. There are two types, one high in mono fats and the other among the highest oil sources of PUFAs. The monounsaturated variety is more prevalent for cooking because of its higher smoke point. It is often blended with canola, making it cheaper to produce, and is often used in salad dressings because it doesn't congeal when refrigerated. The polyunsaturated variety has an extremely high Omega-6 to Omega-3 ratio (133:1 (74% Omega-9), is more prone to going rancid and should not be used in high-heat cooking.

Many people are allergic or hypersensitive to plants of the Asteracese or Compositae family such as daisy, ragweed, marigolds and chrysanthemums. Consumers allergic to these plants may also experience allergic reactions to safflower oil. Some research suggests that safflower oil is toxic to the liver.[57] Since safflower oil is commonly taken for medicinal purposes as a nutritional supplement, many of the warnings that appear on the internet apply to larger and consistent dosing with safflower oil rather than to its occasional use in cooking.

Sesame Oil

(13% Saturated; 42% Monounsaturated; 45% Polyunsaturated)

A traditional ingredient in many types of Asian and Indian cooking, sesame oil is made from the flowering plants of the Sesamun genus. Long used as medicinal oil, it is considered the oldest oilseed crop known to man. It contains high amounts of Vitamin E and is one of the most stable natural oils, but sesame oil can still benefit from refrigeration and limited exposure to light. Cold pressed varieties, while more expensive, are the least processed and retain the most nutrients.

Soybean Oil

(15% Saturated; 61% polyunsaturated; 24% monounsaturated)

Soybean oil is now so ubiquitous in fast foods and processed foods that an astounding 20 percent of the calories in the American diet are estimated to come from this single source. A full discussion of soybeans as a genetically modified crop can be found in Chapter 8, but for purposes here you should know that soybean oil contains high levels of glysophate, the broad spectrum herbicide developed by Monsanto. Most soybean oil will be partially hydrogenated and therefore will contain Trans fats.

Sunflower Oil

(10% Saturated; 20% Monounsaturated; 65% Polyunsaturated)

Food manufacturers have begun to use sunflower oil in popular snack foods in an effort to lower the levels of Trans fats in commercial foods. Refined sunflower oil has an extremely high smoke point (425 F) and is commonly used for commercial frying. It is liquid at room temperature.

If you are already taking a blood thinner for the purpose of decreasing blood clots, sunflower oil may increase the risk of bleeding.

Fake Fats

Olestra

The "ultimate techno-food," according to nutritionist Marion Nestle, is Olestra, the fake fat recently approved by the FDA. Marketed under the brand name Olean, it was approved by the FDA over the objection of dozens of leading scientists.

The additive may be fat-free, but it has a decidedly unhealthy side-effect: it attaches to valuable nutrients and flushes them out of the body. Some of these nutrients, called carotenoids, appear to offer us protection from such diseases as lung cancer, prostate cancer, heart disease, and macular degeneration. Dr. Meir Stampfer, professor of epidemiology at the Harvard School of Public Health, thinks that "the long-term consumption of olestra snack foods might therefore result in several thousand unnecessary deaths each year from lung and prostate cancers and heart disease, and hundreds of additional cases of blindness in the elderly due to macular degeneration. Besides contributing to disease, olestra causes diarrhea and other serious gastrointestinal problems, even at low doses."[58]

The FDA certified Olestra despite such objections and despite the fact that there are already safe, low-fat snacks on the market. There is no evidence to show that Olestra will have any significant effect on reducing obesity in America.

Despite being approved as safe by the FDA, all snacks containing Olestra must carry a warning label with this statement:

This Product Contains Olestra. Olestra may cause abdominal cramping and loose stools. Olestra inhibits the absorption of some vitamins and other nutrients. Vitamins A, D, E, and K have been added.

The Center for Science in the Public Interest has urged food manufacturers to forego olestra and advised consumers to avoid all olestra foods.

Salatrim

This manufactured fat was developed by Nabisco. It has the physical properties of regular fat, but the manufacturer claims it provides only about 5/9 as many calories. Its use can enable companies to make reduced-calorie claims on their products. Salatrim's low calorie content results from its content of stearic acid, which the manufacturer says is absorbed poorly, and short-chain fatty acids, which provide fewer calories per unit weight.

Critics have charged that it does not provide as big a calorie reduction as the manufacturer claims and that only very limited testing has been done to determine effects on humans. Eating small amounts of salatrim is probably safe, but large amounts (30g or more per day) may increase the risk of such side effects as stomach cramps and nausea. No tests have been done to determine if the various food additives (salatrim, olestra, mannitol, and sorbitol) that cause gastrointestinal symptoms can act together to cause greater effects.

Nabisco declared Salatrim safe and has marketed it, as the law allows, without formal FDA approval. (Nabisco has since sold salatrim to another company, Cultor.) In June 1998, the CSPI urged the FDA to ban salatrim until better tests were done and demonstrated safety. Fortunately, salatrim is not widely used.

Eating in the Meantime

- Accepting the "new" reality that saturated fats are not bad for us is not a license to eat bacon at every meal. Fats are still the most energy-dense nutrient. But armed with this knowledge we can better assess those processed foods that brag about being "low fat," and do our best to avoid shortening, margarine, highly refined and hydrogenated oils and those processed foods high in dangerous Trans fats.

- In restaurants that don't have nutrition information readily available, steer clear of fried foods, biscuits, and other baked goods, unless you know that the restaurant has eliminated Trans fat. Many already have, and more will, as we make our voices heard.

- Remember that most commercial vegetable oils contain very little Omega-3 and large amounts of the Omega-6 fatty acids.

- Whenever possible, buy oils in glass containers, not pliable plastic which leaches the solvent toluene into the contents.

- When you fry, use butter, or a fully saturated fat like lard, or coconut oil. Bake with butter, coconut oil, olive oil and other heat stable oils. Frankly, they taste better anyway.

- Unfortunately, many of the most healthful oils are also the most expensive. Consider sharing the purchase of these oils with a friend or neighbor

- Until further research confirms the safety of Olestra, parents shouldn't take the chance on this highly controversial fake fat. Olestra is currently used almost exclusively in the manufacture of "low fat" potato chips. You and your kids can live without these. Look for the Trans fat listing on the Nutrition Facts label. Compare brands and choose the one lowest in Trans fat.

Chapter 6. Meaty Problems

For many Americans, meat is the centerpiece of every meal. We eat more of it than any country on earth—about one-sixth of global consumption, although we comprise only about one-twentieth of the world's population. We've long been a nation of meat-eaters, and red meat eaters at that. Americans eat more than 60 pounds of cow annually, and red meat still represents the largest proportion (58%) of meat consumed in the US.

We're starting to cut back a little. While meat consumption increased significantly over the last century, nearly doubling between 1909 and 2007,[59] for the first time in almost two decades that trend is changing. We're eating more poultry in relation to red meat now, and more pork. But we still eat more meat per person than any almost anywhere else on earth. Over 200 pounds per person per year.

I think it's a good thing that American consumers are eating less meat. There are plenty of health benefits to reducing, or eliminating, meat from the diet. But if you're expecting a polemic on vegetarianism, you won't find it here. We evolved as hunters and gatherers long before agriculture. We share physiological characteristics of both carnivores and omnivores. While it's perfectly possibly to be healthy on a strictly vegetarian diet, meat has been part of the balance for humans for millennia, and it's not likely to disappear from the dinner plate anytime soon.

From a health standpoint the problem is not so much what meat is, but what is done to it in the highly mechanized modern systems that take our meat from insemination to slaughter to table.

Drugging Our Meat

One consequence of the mechanization of our meat supply has been the wholesale practice of drugging our meat. Cattle, swine and poultry are routinely given antimicrobials throughout much of their lives. These are the same wonder drugs that protect humans from bacterial infections, but the bulk of these drugs—over 80%—are administered to livestock, not people. This massive overuse in animal agriculture has led to the evolution of antibiotic-resistant bacteria, increasing the risk of deadly infections in humans that are difficult and costly to treat.

Antibiotics

For at least the last half century meat producers have been dosing their animals, and by extension, those of us who eat them, with low levels of antibiotics like penicillin and tetracycline. The motivation for this "sub-therapeutic" dosing of antibiotics is growth promotion. Treated animals gain much more weight than they otherwise would, and those extra pounds mean extra profit for producers.

The practice, however, has long raised concerns about serious health risks and human drug resistance. In the 1970s, the FDA asked producers to show that their use of penicillin and tetracycline caused no harm to humans. When they couldn't, the agency banned the use of the drugs in animals. But under pressure from the drug and animal industries, Congress stepped in and ordered the FDA not to implement the ban.

In 1999, and again in 2005, petitions were filed by the Center for Science in the Public Interest, Environmental Defense, the American Academy of Pediatrics, the American Public Health Association, Food Animal Concerns Trust (FACT), and the Union of Concerned Scientists. Both petitions had asked the agency to withdrawal its approval of certain antimicrobial drugs that are considered important for human medicine. In June 2010, the FDA finally admitted that antibiotics in meat pose a "serious public health threat," but despite this admission, the agency denied both petitions. Instead, the agency asked producers to voluntarily use the drugs "judiciously" with the oversight of a veterinarian. In 2011, the agency asked pharmaceutical companies to voluntarily reduce sales of antibiotics for use in food animals. The industry response? Sales of the two most commonly used antibiotics in livestock and poultry increased for the second consecutive year.

For a vast number of scientists, health experts, and public interest groups, saying "pretty please" to livestock producers and drug companies is just not enough. Legislation has been pending in Congress since 2013 that would address this problem. *The Preservation of Antibiotics for Medical Treatment Act* (PAMTA, H.R. 965, S. 1211) would withdraw the routine use of seven classes of antibiotics vitally important to human health from food animal production unless the animals are sick or unless drug companies can prove that their use does not harm human health.

Nearly every major medical organization in the US supports PAMTA, including the American Medical Association, American Academy of Pediatricians, Infectious Diseases Society of America, the American Nurses Association and the World Health Organization. Cities across the US passed resolutions to encourage Congress to pass PAMTA and consumer rights organizations have collected thousands of signatures. Still, Congress refused to act.

> Putting an end to the involuntary dosing of meat-eating Americans with antibiotics may well be the most critical battle in the Great American Food Fight.

Putting an end to the involuntary dosing of meat-eating Americans with antibiotics may well be the most critical battle in the Great American Food Fight. The number of cases of antibiotic-resistant infections (ABRs) has more than doubled over the past decade, costing the US healthcare system over $20 billion annually, and already killing more Americans each year than AIDS. This is an avoidable national health crisis, but the FDA refuses to act. The use of sub-therapeutic antibiotics in meat animals has already been banned in many countries in the European Union and in Canada. Our own FDA needs to do the same.

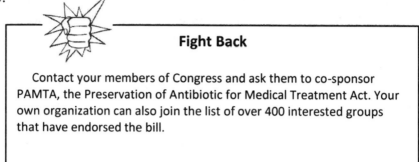

Fight Back

Contact your members of Congress and ask them to co-sponsor PAMTA, the Preservation of Antibiotic for Medical Treatment Act. Your own organization can also join the list of over 400 interested groups that have endorsed the bill.

Ractopamine

Another drug used to fatten the bottom line is ractopamine hydrochloride, used for boosting the growth of swine and pigs in the last weeks before slaughter. Fed to an estimated 60 to 80% of US pigs, it also causes meat to have a higher water content which effectively penalizes the consumer.

Ractopamine belongs to the class of beta-adrenoceptor agonists, drugs which bind to beta-receptors in the heart, causing systemic dilation of blood vessels. Drugs like ractopamine can cause restlessness, anxiety, rapid heart rate, and other conditions. It was approved in 1999 based on animal studies submitted by the drug's manufacturer. The single human study included only six men, one of whom was removed because his heart began racing and pounding abnormally.[60]

No long term studies have been conducted to determine the safety or the effects of ractopamine hydrochloride in humans, and no data exists relating to the long-term exposure of humans to the chemical. A 2009 European Food Safety Authority evaluation concluded that no acceptable daily intake for ractopamine could be established.[61] As of this writing, 160 countries, including China, Russia, and the European Union, have banned the use of ractopamine.

Steroids and Growth Hormones

There are currently six different kinds of steroid hormones that are approved by the FDA for use in food production. Estradiol and progesterone, which are natural female sex hormones; testosterone, the natural male sex hormone; and three synthetic hormone-like chemicals are allowed to make cattle and sheep grow faster. Federal regulations don't allow these hormones to be used on poultry or hogs, perhaps because they have not been found to be extremely useful in increasing weight gain in these animals. Estrogen, however, may still be introduced into chicken feed in the form of soy protein and animal protein meal.

Given the fact that most Americans have been eating hormone-dosed beef for over fifty years, it's remarkable that so little research has been done to assess possible health risks. The minimal research available and the simple biologic *plausibility* of health implications has been enough for the European Union and Canada to make the practice illegal in meat production in these countries. The EU has gone so far as to ban the import of US beef and dairy from treated animals.

For now, no conclusive evidence exists either to support or totally refute the purported health risks from consuming meat from hormonally treated cows. We do know, however, that too much of any hormone can disrupt human hormone balance, causing developmental problems, interfering with the reproductive system, and even leading to the development of breast,[62] prostate and colon cancers. We know that the highest rates of hormone-dependent cancer, such as cancer of the breast, endometrium, ovary, prostate, testes, and colon, are found in North America. We know that maternal beef consumption is associated with lower sperm concentration and possible sub fertility.[63] And the connection between hormones in food and the alarming rise in precocious puberty, especially in girls, has gone well beyond suspicious. [64, 65]

Human exposure to endocrine disrupting chemicals is abundant in the environment as well as in our food. We've already discussed their presence in plastics and packaging. Hormones in meat and animal feed may not be the chief cause of this explosion in reproductive and childhood cancers, but they are surely adding to the problem.

In 2010 several scientists, including Dr. Samuel S. Epstein, cancer prevention expert and Professor emeritus of Environmental & Occupational Medicine at the University of Illinois School of Public Health in Chicago, petitioned the FDA for an urgent ban on hormonal meat. Of particular concern, says Epstein, are the increased risks of hormonal cancers since 1975: breast by 23%, prostate by 60%, and testes by 60%. The petition warns that the ban on hormonal meat is three decades overdue and that the use of sex hormones to increase meat production poses imminent hazards to the total U.S. population.

Despite international scientific concern, the United States, backed by the World Trade Organization, continues to allow growth-promoting hormones in cattle. Meat is not monitored for sex hormone levels by the USDA or FDA.

Meat Fillers and Extenders

While cattle inventory in the US has dropped in recent decades, we are still producing more beef now than we did in the 1970s. This apparent contradiction can be explained by the success of farmers and corporate scientists who have found ways to get more meat out of every cow. There are a surprising number of ways to "stretch" meat. While we consumers are happy to have affordable meat, we are rarely aware that we are buying non-meat, and sometimes indigestible, fillers.

Meat extenders are non-meat substances with substantial protein content. These usually consist of a cereal mixture combined with meat, fat, blood and internal organs and are common in processed meats such as hot dogs and breakfast sausages.

Fillers, on the other hand, are normally high in carbohydrates and may contain the combinations of flours and oatmeal that are often used in hot dogs. Other common fillers include bread crumbs and maltodextrin, a food additive made from starch, and soya protein, a common ingredient in cheap hamburgers. All are used primarily for making meat products less expensive.

In addition to extenders and fillers of non-meat origin, the cheaper, mechanically separated parts from animal carcasses, also known as **mechanically deboned meats (MDM***)*, are widely used in meat processing, especially in poultry processing. Formed chicken products, like chicken nuggets, usually contain MDM, as well as a high percentage of non-meat fillers, like corn, along with twenty or thirty other ingredients.

Pink Slime

Pink slime is the term used for a mixture of beef scraps and connective tissue (formerly used only for pet food and rendering) that is treated with ammonia hydroxide to remove pathogens like salmonella and E coli. These so-called "Lean Beef Trimmings," have been used in beef products since the 1990s, but in 2011, when celebrity chef Jamie Oliver used his television show and social media to alert the public to its presence, especially in school lunches, the slime hit the fan.

Due to public outcry, fast food giants like McDonald's and Burger King have stopped using pink slime in their food. Grocers, too, are responding to disgusted consumers and promising not to sell pink slime in beef products, and the FDA has been forced to back off its whole-hearted endorsement of the ammonia-treated filler.

Not everyone thinks that the pink slime uproar resulted in a major victory for consumers in the Great American Food Fight. Even the Center for Science in the Public Interest found it a "tempest in a teapot," given what else goes into our food. But the episode definitely demonstrated how fast change can come when informed consumers raise their voices together. The "pink slime" coverage significantly changed ground beef in the U.S. Several manufacturing plants were shuttered after public backlash and, according to industry officials, the ammonia-treated filler is now used only in an estimated 5% of our beef, down from 70% at its peak use in 2012. The FDA, however, still insists that pink slime is safe and continues to order it for the National School Lunch Program.

Cellulose, Meat Glue, and More

Meat glue is composed of an enzyme called transglutaminase (TG) which is used to stick together chunks of meat that are too small to sell. Some meat glues are laboratory produced through the cultivation of bacteria, while others are made from the coagulant in the blood of pigs and cows. Neither food manufacturers nor restaurants are required to inform you that they've glued your meat together, but if transglutaminase is used in a product, it must be identified on the ingredients label as "TG enzyme," "enzyme" or "TGP enzyme." Meats containing transglutaminase will be labeled as "formed" or "reformed," as in "formed beef tenderloin," or "reformed beef tenderloin pieces."

A recent spate of publicity has surrounded the potential dangers of transglutaminase to those who suffer from celiac disease. In celiac disease, our systems make antibodies to our own tissue transglutaminase enzyme, causing our immune systems to attack our intestinal linings. Some experts claim that the enzyme in meat glue is not the same as that in our bodies. Others argue that the molecule will behave exactly the same way regardless of where it's produced. Complicating the problem is the fact that some formulations of commercial meat glue do contain wheat, MSG, or milk casein, all of which may pose dangers to those with celiac disease.

Bacterial contamination of meat-glued steak is hundreds of times higher than a solid piece of steak; therefore, if you cook your steak rare, which is ordinarily the most healthful way to cook your meat, you're at a much greater risk of contracting food poisoning.

While you might not expect to find wood pulp in your food, it's often there, in the form of powdered or gummed **cellulose**. Indeed, the use of cellulose as a food additive has exploded in the last decade as more and more producers are finding it a cost-saving filler or binder for processed foods. As an added bonus, manufacturers can eliminate fat from foods and also get to brag about added "all natural" fiber.

Humans are unable to digest cellulose because we lack the appropriate enzymes to break it down, but, like other fibers, it can aid in the smooth working of the intestinal tract. Many consumers, however, given the choice, would prefer a nutritive fiber. The USDA, which regulates meats, has set a limit of 3.5% on the use of cellulose in meat.

Salt Water

In a practice called "plumping," manufacturers inject saltwater into raw meat, especially chicken, to enhance flavor and increase the weight of the meat before it's sold. Meat that's been injected with saltwater may say "flavored with up to 10% of a solution" or "up to 15% chicken broth." Regular chicken has about 40 to 70 mg of sodium per 4-ounce serving, while plumped chicken can contain 5 times or more than that amount, or 300 mg and up. Consumers on low sodium diets should check the fine print and the nutrition facts label.

Grass Fed vs. Corn Fed

While ruminant, or cud-chewing, animals are built to eat plants, most production cattle since World War II has been fed corn. The corn diet allows them to be fed in Confined Animal Feeding Operations, (CAFOs) where as many as 100,000 cattle may live in their own manure. It also facilities the administration of the hormones and antibiotics we've discussed.

"Grass fed" is commonly understood to mean meat from animals that graze in open pastures, not those raised in feedlots. The grass fed label is FDA regulated now. It means that the animals cannot be fed grain or grain by-products and must have continuous access to pasture during the growing season. But it almost didn't. The USDA had originally proposed a voluntary 80% grass-fed standard. Many groups, including Consumers Union, objected. In a rare win for consumers, the

USDA withdrew that proposed standard.

The science is confirming that these grass-fed animals provide significant health benefits over feedlot finished livestock. A recent analysis from the Union of Concerned Scientists found that grass-fed steak has about twice as many Omega-3s as a typical grain-fed steak. In another study published in March 2010 in *Nutrition Journal*, researchers supported those numbers, also finding higher concentrations of vitamin E and other antioxidants in grass-fed beef.[66]

Unfortunately, the grass-fed label does not limit the use of antibiotics, hormones, or pesticides. To be sure that the meat you buy comes from animals that were raised without antibiotics or growth hormones, look for the "Certified Humane Raised & Handled" label. The label, which is partially funded by the American Society for the Prevention of Cruelty to Animals, also mandates animal-care standards.

Meat and Mortality

Until recently the research on meat and mortality has been ambiguous or contradictory. With the 2012 publication of two of the largest studies of red-meat consumption and premature death ever undertaken, the picture has cleared. Two major Harvard studies which followed more than 120,000 American men and women for up to 22 years found that red meat consumption was associated with living a significantly shorter life.[67,68] Even after factoring out lifestyle risks and known contributors of disease, meat consumption was still linked to increased cancer mortality, increased heart disease mortality, and increased overall mortality. The study's authors concluded that replacing one serving per day of red meat with an alternative like fish, legumes, or poultry was associated with around 10% decreased mortality risk. Replacing one serving per day of processed red meat was associated with around 20% decreased mortality risk.

> **What exactly is in the meat that is so significantly increasing cancer death rates, heart disease, and shortening people's lives?**
>
> A few possibilities include heme iron, nitrosamines, biogenic amines, advanced glycation end products, arachidonic acid, steroids, toxic metals, drug residues, viruses, heterocyclic amines, PCBs, dioxins, and other industrial pollutants.
>
> **Source: Michael Greger, M.D.**

Hot Dogs and Other Processed Meat

Processed meats are those that have been preserved by curing, smoking, salting, or adding chemical preservatives, and here the research is much less ambiguous. Studies have linked the consumption of processed meats to adult colorectal cancer,[69] renal cancer,[70] stomach cancers,[71] pancreatic cancer, bladder cancers,[72] heart disease and diabetes.[73]

Twenty-two percent of the meat consumed in the U.S. is processed. What virtually all of that processed meat has in common is the additive, sodium nitrite.

Nitrates and Nitrites

Nitrites and nitrates are among the class of chemicals called *nitrosamines* that are created by a chemical reaction between nitrites or other proteins. The vast majority of nitrosamines are known carcinogens and the presence of nitrites and nitrates in food has concerned health authorities for decades. In the 1970's the USDA actually tried to ban this additive but was vetoed by food manufacturers who complained they had no alternative for preserving packaged meat products.

Sodium *nitrite* is a salty preservative used to delay the development of botulism in processed meats. The chemical imparts a cured meat flavor, but it also turns the product bright red, suggesting freshness to most consumers. Sodium *nitrate* is a natural antioxidant found in leafy vegetables. Both chemicals form nitrosamines, but vegetables also contain ascorbic acid (Vitamin C) and alpha tocopherol (Vitamin E) which inhibit nitrosamine formation. Both of these vitamins may be added to cured meats to inhibit nitrosamine formation.

The favorite processed meat of children, of course, is the all American hot dog. The science, however, suggests that there may be good reason to put some limits on this favorite food, for kids and for expectant parents, too.

In studying the relationship between the intake of certain foods and the risk of leukemia in children, a California team found that children eating more than 12 hot dogs per month had nine times the normal risk of developing childhood leukemia. A strong risk for childhood leukemia also existed for those children whose fathers' intake of hot dogs was 12 or more per month.[74]

Researchers Sarusua and Savitz studied childhood cancer cases in Denver and found that children born to mothers who consumed hot dogs one or more times per week during pregnancy had approximately double the risk of developing brain tumors. Children who ate hot dogs one or more times per week were also at higher risk of brain cancer.[75] Bunin et al, also found that maternal consumption of hot dogs during pregnancy was associated with an excess risk of childhood brain tumors.[76]

As with so many of the chemicals we eat directly, exposure is compounded in the environment, too. Nitrates and nitrites are widely found in fertilizers, pesticides and cosmetics. Nitrate contents in drinking water may also contribute considerably to human exposure.

Nitrate may be labeled *sodium nitrate*, *nitrite* or *sodium nitrites*, and all of these should be limited. Nitrate-free hot dogs and deli meats are becoming available, but you'll have to read the label. Celery juice powder is also being used as an organic replacement for sodium nitrite.

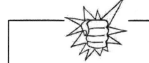

Fight Back!

Write the FDA to express your concern that nitrite-hot dogs are not labeled for their cancer risk to children. You can mention the Cancer Prevention Coalition's petition on hot dogs, docket #: 95P 0112/CP1

Chicken and Poultry

As beef consumption began to decline in the 1970s, poultry consumption rose quickly. The last few years have seen chicken surpass beef as our No. 1 meat of choice. The switch to chicken may eliminate the risks of the endocrine disrupting chemicals present in beef, but antibiotics are also used in production poultry to ensure large, fast-growing birds. It's a system, apparently, that works astonishingly well. According to the University of Arkansas Division of Agriculture, if we grew as fast as a chicken, we'd weigh 349 pounds at age 2.

In many cases, chickens receive antibiotic drugs from the time that they are in the egg all the way up to the time they are slaughtered. These chemicals are also found in high concentrations in their feces, which means that fecal pollution from chicken farms is especially disastrous for the environment.

But fecal contamination can also get as far as your table. An independent laboratory test commissioned by Physicians for

Responsible Medicine in 2012 found fecal contamination in 48% of the samples collected from 15 different grocery chains in 10 major cities. The findings suggest that skinless chicken is at least as likely as to be contaminated as chicken with skin left intact. Likewise, antibiotic-free products appear to be as likely as "conventional" chicken to be contaminated. Nearly 50 percent of both types of products tested positive for fecal traces. [77]

Chicken is an incredibly versatile meat food. It's an excellent source of protein and of several important vitamins and antioxidants, including B6, Niacin and Selenium. But to limit our exposure to antibiotics and other chemicals, we'll have to pay more.

Organic Poultry

To qualify for the USDA organic seal, poultry must be raised organically no later than two days after hatching and cannot be grown using persistent pesticides or chemical fertilizers. Birds must never be fed animal by-products or genetically engineered grains. No antibiotics or other drugs may be administered to them. USDA regulations also mandate that chicken, labeled "organic" must be allowed access to the outside, direct sunlight, fresh air and freedom of movement."

Free Range and Cage Free

The vaguely defined **free range** label is also an FDA designation, but it does not address food sources or chemicals. The label requires that animals have the ability to access the outdoors without specifying the amount of daily time this entails or the size of the outdoor space. In reality, the care of free range hens may be so structured that the hens are very unlikely to go outside.

The **cage free** designation simply means that the hens are not kept in traditional battery cages—the 67 square inch boxes in which hens may live their entire lives. The European Union has already phased out battery cages. Californians have voted to ban them as of 2015. Other states have legislation pending.

Under current regulatory language, all organic chickens are free-range, but all free-range chicken is not necessarily <u>organic.</u> The only way to be certain you're avoiding antibiotics, GE feed, and other chemicals and to at least reduce the risk of fecal contamination is to buy 100% Certified Organic poultry. The birds may cost twice as much, and they will be paler in color and much smaller, but you'll be buying safer and healthier meat.

Fish and Seafood

The heart-protective effects of eating fish and seafood have been observed for decades in native populations in Alaska and Greenland and among the fish-loving Japanese. Evidence continues to indicate that eating fish once a week may significantly reduce CHD.[78] There is also limited but suggestive evidence that fish consumption reduces the risk of breast, colorectal and prostate cancers.

Fish benefits would seem to outweigh the risks, but that doesn't mean there aren't any.

PCBs

Polychlorinated biphenyls (PCBs) are toxic industrial compounds that were banned in 1979, but that persist in the environment. Fish absorb PCBs from contaminated sediments and from their food. Unlike mercury, which is more quickly eliminated from the body, PCBs are stored in body fat for many years, but you can limit exposure to PCBs simply by trimming, skinning and cooking your catch to reduce fatty tissue.

Mercury

In 2004, the EPA and the FDA issued a joint advisory about mercury in fish for pregnant women, women who might become pregnant, nursing mothers, and children. The following three recommendations are still in effect.

- Do not eat shark, swordfish, king mackerel, or tilefish because they contain high levels of mercury.

- Eat up to 12 ounces (two average meals) each week of a variety of fish and shellfish that are lower in mercury.

  - Five of the most commonly consumed fish that are low in mercury are shrimp, canned light tuna, salmon, pollock, and catfish.
  - Albacore ("white") tuna is another commonly consumed fish that has more mercury than canned, light tuna. Eat up to 6 ounces (one average meal) of albacore tuna per week.

- Check local advisories about the safety of fish caught by family and friends in local lakes, rivers, and coastal areas. If no advice is available, eat up to 6 ounces (one average meal) per week of fish caught from local waters, but do not consume any other fish during that week.

Follow these same recommendations when including fish and shellfish in a young child's diet, but serve smaller portions.[79]

No Organic Fish

The USDA does not currently provide organic standards for fish and shellfish, so seafood labeled "organic" is not only deceptive, but it may still contain contaminants like PCBs and mercury. You'll have to rely on other sources for assurance that seafood is low in contaminants or was caught using sustainable practices.

Seafood Safe, a voluntary fish-labeling program for companies, retailers and restaurants, uses the EPA guidelines to identify seafood with safe consumption levels of mercury and PCBs. Businesses displaying the label have undergone a confidential pre-assessment and are subject to customized testing regimes.

Three non-profits also publish fish advisory cards on the Web. Visit these websites:

The Monterrey Bay Aquarium: (www.montereybayaquarium.org),
The Blue Ocean Institute (www.blueocean.org), and
Environmental Defense (www.environmentaldefense.org) for cell phone aps and pocket seafood guides.

Genetically Modified Fish

In 2015 The Food and Drug Administration approved the application by Aqua Bounty Farms to permit sales of genetically engineered salmon for commercial production, sale and consumption, making the GE salmon the first genetically modified animal to enter the human food supply. The human health impacts of eating GE fish are entirely unknown, but ecological and ethical concerns also motivated the more than 20 anti-GMO organizations who opposed the FDA move. The next phase of the battle, whether GMO fish will be labeled, giving consumers the ability to identify the new "frankenfish" in supermarkets, is still ahead. See Chapter 8 for a discussion of the fight for GMO labeling in fish and other foods.

Meat Substitutes

The most popular meat substitutes are soy products. Tofu, of course, is a staple of Western vegetarian cooking and almost a synonym for vegetarianism itself. Here, however, are some meat alternatives you may not know about. One is still on the drawing board. The other is already in the supermarket.

In vitro meat

While it may sound a lot like a bad sci-fi movie, lab-grown meat may be coming to a supermarket near you. In vitro meat, also known as cultured meat, is an animal flesh product that has never been part of a complete, living animal. Several current research projects are growing *in vitro* meat experimentally, although no meat has yet been produced for public consumption.

The first-generation products will most likely be minced meat, and a long-term goal is to grow fully developed muscle tissue. In 2008, People for the Ethical Treatment of Animals (PETA) announced a contest offering a $1 million dollar prize to the contestant who can make the first commercially available in vitro chicken meat.[80] About 30 labs around the world, including several in the U.S., have announced work on in vitro meat.

The thought of lab-grown meat, for now, may sound unappetizing, but the prospect of satisfying the world's meat hunger without animal cruelty and with less environmental impact is an idea well worth chewing on.

Mycoprotein

While you've likely never ordered *Fusarium venenatum*, you may have eaten it. It's processed mold, the novel ingredient in Quorn-brand frozen meat substitutes. Manufactured by Marlow Foods in Marlow, England, where the organism from which it is grown was first discovered in the soil.

Quorn foods are labeled as "mushroom protein" or "mushroom in origin," but the mold, actually the fungus, from which it is made, does not produce mushrooms. Rather, the mold is grown in liquid solution in large tanks. It has been sold in the United Kingdom since the 1990s and marketed in the United States since 2002.

On the positive side, mycoprotein is nutritious and low in sodium. It doesn't require the land, water, and energy resources required of beef and poultry production. Of course, it's vegetarian, and many consumers think it does, indeed, "taste just like chicken." But consumption of Quorn products have caused allergic reactions and gastrointestinal distress in some people, with symptoms resulting in vomiting, nausea, diarrhea, and, less often, hives and potentially fatal anaphylactic reactions.[81] A UK survey sponsored by the CSPI found that the percentage of consumers sensitive to Quorn is probably as great as, or greater than, the percentage sensitive to soy, milk, peanuts, and other common food allergens.

The British and American governments acknowledge that Quorn foods may cause allergic reactions, but so far both have rejected the CSPI's recommendations to prohibit the use of mycoprotein or at least to require Quorn foods to bear a warning label. In fact, when Quorn-containing "vegetarian" products are served at restaurants, cafeterias, and other foodservice locations, there is no label to let consumers know that they are eating Quorn foods.

On frozen processed foods sold in the US, the term *Mycoprotein*, or the company trademark (Quorn™) will be listed in the ingredients list at the bottom of the Nutrition Facts panel. Consumers who believe they have been sickened by Quorn foods may file a report with the Center for Science in the Public Interest.

Ethical and Environmental Issues

Authors and investigative journalists like Michael Pollan (*The Omnivore's Dilemma, In Defense of Food, etc.*) and Eric Schlossser *(Fast Food Nation)* have raised the consciousness of American consumers about the facts, and some of the horrors, of industrialized meat production and how much it has changed in a very short time. The centralization of the meat industry, driven by the large fast food chains, has resulted in fewer and fewer suppliers to bigger slaughterhouses, bigger processing facilities, and really big meatpacking companies.

There are obviously many ethical issues that arise from how animals are treated in these huge and complex systems. We've touched on only a few of them. But the quality of the environment also influences the quality and safety of foods and here especially our hunger for plentiful, cheap meat may be costing more than we realize. Livestock production alone contributes to 18 percent of the global warming effect—more than the emissions from every single car, train, and plane on the planet. Though livestock production only contributes 9 percent of carbon dioxide emissions, the sector is responsible for 37 percent of methane and 65 percent of nitrous oxide, both potent greenhouse gases.

Meat production is also having a serious impact on the under-developed world, where ancient rain forests are being cleared to provide land for cattle grazing or feed grains. These practices are resulting in less available land for other food, more global warming, and depletion of the world's water supplies. They are also contributing to an expanding need for foreign aid and to growing world hunger.

The consumption of meat is taking a toll on the health of the world's poorest people as well as on its wealthiest consumers. While vegetarianism may be a bridge too far for many of us, there are abundant economic, ethical, and health reasons to cut back, even a little, on meat.

What about Protein?

The big concern for individuals or families who are considering vegetarianism or a significant reduction in meat consumption is whether they'll be getting enough protein. Our protein worries, however, are largely misplaced. Protein deficiencies are rare in developed countries and most Americans, including vegetarians, eat much more than we need. In general, it's recommended that 10–35% of your daily calories come from protein. A chart showing the Recommended Dietary Allowances of protein for different age groups and alternative sources of protein can be found in the Appendix.

Driving Range

Substituting chicken, fish, or eggs for red meat and dairy just one day a week for a year would reduce greenhouse gas emissions by an amount equivalent to not driving 760 miles. Going completely vegetarian one day a week for a year is equivalent to not driving 1,160 miles.

Source: Environ. Sci. Techno. 42: 3508.2008.

Rather than just focusing on your protein needs, choose an overall healthy eating plan that provides the protein you need as well as other nutrients.

Eating in the Meantime

- The healthiest approach for non-vegetarians is avoiding factory farmed raised livestock as much as possible. Eat a little less meat, ideally organic and local, more fish, and plenty of plant based foods.

- When you need ground meat, consider selecting your own cuts of meat and having your butcher grind it in front of you. Your burgers will be more expensive, but they won't contain head meat, internal organs, fillers, or extenders. An extended discussion of Recombinant Bovine Growth Hormone (rBGH) as it is used in dairy cattle for milk production appears in Chapter 7. This hormone is not used on beef cattle.

- For pork raised without antibiotics or ractopamine, buy Certified Organic. U.S. food companies which avoid meat produced with the feed additive ractopamine include Chipotle restaurants, meat producer Niman Ranch, and Whole Foods Markets.

- Children and potential parents should not consume 12 or more hot dogs per month. Read nutrition labels on other processed meats to see how much additional nitrite may be in other sources.

- Request that your supermarket stock nitrite-free hot dogs. Most stores will be happy to comply. If they refuse, take your grocery ballot elsewhere.

- Contact your local school board to inquire about whether your children are being served hot dogs containing nitrite in the cafeteria.

- Remember that "all-natural," "free-range" or "hormone-free" product labels on poultry do not mean that these birds have been fed organic feed or given access to the outdoors.

- Don't succumb to thinking of vegetarianism as an "either/or" proposition. If you'd like to reduce meat consumption in your household, start with a meatless Monday. Be weekday vegetarians. Or weekend vegetarians. Support family members, especially teens, who take a principled stand on vegetarianism.

- When you reduce the amount of meat that goes on your grocery list ballot, you're voting for a safer, greener planet, less animal cruelty, and a healthier family. Bonus: You're also saving money!

Chapter 7. Milking the Public: What's in the Dairy Case?

Got milk? If you're a US citizen, your government certainly hopes so. It runs massive educational and marketing campaigns to convince you and your children to drink it, and bears much of the cost for seeing that it's in school lunches. It's paying farmers to produce it, protecting them from international price competition, even promising to buy back from processors any amount of cheese, butter, or nonfat dry milk that you don't buy.

As do most of our farm policies, dairy subsidies cost the US taxpayer dearly. The tab has run to about $40 billion in the last ten years, $222 million in 2012 alone. Dairy subsidies add millions of dollars to the grocery bills of American consumers and to the costs of food product manufacturers, while benefitting only a relative handful of large farmers. In fact, 62 percent of US farmers collect no subsidy payments at all.

Our national dairy policy is complex, inequitable, and extraordinarily expensive. But those may not be its biggest problems. The worst thing about US dairy policy is that it encourages practices that are ultimately detrimental to public health.

The Perfect Food?

Most of us grew up hearing the injunction to "Drink your milk!" at almost every meal. Milk, we understood, was the kid-fuel that made for strong bones, sound teeth, and a passing grade on Mrs. Watson's pop arithmetic quiz. Milk was the nectar of childhood, as beyond reproach as any foodstuff can get.

Today? Not so much. In the last decade or so milk has been rapidly losing fans and acquiring critics. Even the late Dr. Benjamin Spock reversed his support of cow's milk for children in 1998 in his last edition of his world-famous book *Baby and Child Care.*

What's responsible for sullying milk's lily white reputation? How has the sacred cow of the American diet fallen from nutritional grace?

Osteoporosis

For starters, it seems that some of those inviolate truisms that we were taught about milk might not be true after all. Take that one about milk preventing osteoporosis—the bone disease that leads to increased risk of fracture. It turns out that the cause of osteoporosis in later life is not the result of failure to drink our milk, or even to take in enough calcium. It's what we do to deplete our bodies of calcium.

Dr. Neal D. Barnard, president of the Physicians Committee for Responsible Medicine, speaks for a new wave of researchers who are disputing the conventional wisdom on osteoporosis. Barnard maintains that cow's milk is not just unnecessary but harmful, and that the real causes of osteoporosis factors that leach calcium from the bones: animal protein, caffeine, sodium, tobacco, and sedentary lifestyle."[82]

In spite of what we were told as kids, and what the dairy industry would still like us to believe, milk provides little or no benefit to bones. In fact, it may pose a danger. The Harvard Nurses' Health Study, one of the largest investigations ever undertaken into the risk factors for major chronic diseases in women, found that women with the highest calcium consumption from dairy products actually had substantially more fractures than women who drank less milk.[83] Milk doesn't improve bone integrity in children either.[84] In fact, a 2012 study found that, among the most physically active girls, those who got the most calcium from dairy products in their diets had more than double the risk of stress fractures.[85]

The fact that milk doesn't really protect our bones may be only one of the reasons for parents to reconsider whether telling the kids to "Drink Your Milk!" is still such a good idea. Milk's reputation as a great weight loss food may also be undeserved.

The Skinny on Milk and Weight Loss

Since 2004, when a study conducted at the University of Tennessee (and sponsored by the National Dairy Council) compared the effects of three different calorie-restricted diets on weight loss, many consumers have been convinced that drinking higher amounts of milk or eating other dairy foods might help them win the battle of the bulge. The study, which followed only 32 obese adults, showed that all of the groups lost weight, but those who ate the dairy-rich diet lost the most. The study was broadly publicized by the dairy industry which developed extensive marketing campaigns promoting the weight loss benefits of its products. Articles touting milk as a diet food still appear widely on the internet.

The preponderance of research, however, from studies before and after the dairy industry-sponsored 2004 study, simply doesn't bear this out.

An assessment of evidence from 49 clinical trials from 1966 to 2007 showed that neither dairy products nor calcium supplements helped people lose weight. Of the 49 clinical trials, 41 showed no effect, two demonstrated weight gain, one showed a lower rate of weight gain, and only five showed weight loss.[86]

While most of these trials looked at adult subjects, the same results were also found with children. A longitudinal cohort of 12,829 US children, aged 9 to 14, found no weight loss advantages to milk. Children who drank more than 3 servings a day of milk gained more in BMI than those who drank milk in smaller quantities. Skim and 1% milk were associated with weight gain, but dairy fat was not. Children who drank the most milk gained more weight.[87]

Calories obtained from dairy products are certainly more nutritional that sweetened cola drinks, but the evidence does not seem to support the dairy industry's promotion of milk as a diet food.[88]

Milk's reputation as the perfect food is undeserved in more ways than one. Milk doesn't really protect our bones. And unless it substitutes for higher calorie foods in the diet, it won't help us lose weight. But the problems with milk don't stop there. There's a significant difference in the way that milk is produced today. One that makes us, and our children, test subjects in one of the largest, and potentially most dangerous, animal experiment ever conducted.

GMO Milk

The first mass-marketed genetically modified food was milk, containing bovine somatotropin (bST), or recombinant bovine growth hormone (rBGH). A genetic manipulation of bacteria, engineered and patented by Monsanto, the hormone was sold under the trade name Posilac. It is administered to cattle by injection to simulate a naturally occurring hormone (IGF-1) which the cow uses to convert nutrients into milk. The artificial growth hormone works so well that opponents have called it "crack for cows." It can increase milk production by up to 30%.

That kind of boost in milk production had obvious appeal to the dairy industry, but scientists worried about the effect of the increased levels of the insulin-like growth factor IGF-1 on human health. One of the most outspoken of these was Dr. Samuel Epstein from the University of Illinois's School of Public Health. Epstein warned that a mounting body of evidence linked IGF-1 to the development of human cancers. The growth promoting hormone had already been incriminated as a possible cause of breast, colon, and prostate cancers.

Despite such criticism the FDA approved rBGH in 1993. The approval was based solely on one study administered by Monsanto in which rBGH was tested for 90 days on 30 rats. Although the FDA maintains that the results showed no significant problems, the study was never actually published and still remains secret. To this day, Monsanto, with FDA cooperation, has refused to allow anyone outside the administration to examine the data from the study. [89]

Beyond the milking of the American consumer in denying us the scientific scrutiny for which the FDA presumably exists, its approval of rBGH set in motion other dangerous precedents for which we're still paying the costs.

By the early nineties, and despite Monsanto's numerous public assurances to the contrary, it became apparent that all those hormone injections were pretty brutal on the cows. Hormone-treated animals developed serious health problems. They suffered from higher incidences of deformed births as well as udder infections and lameness, which demanded treatment with antibiotics. A solution came quickly, from a former chief scientist for Monsanto. In her new position as Deputy Director of Human Food Safety for the FDA, Dr. Margaret Miller raised the standard for permissible levels of antibiotics in milk by 100 times over the existing standard. She deserves considerable credit for the drugging of our national meat and milk supply and for the alarming rise in antibiotic-resistant bacteria we're experiencing today.

Another decision surrounding the new hormone, which would bear heavily on public health as well as Monsanto's profits, was also made about the same time. Under the guidance of former Monsanto lawyer Michael R. Taylor in his new position of Deputy Commissioner for Policy, the FDA decided not to label GMO foods.[90]

Two decades later, the struggle to label GMO foods wages on. In our own country the massive human experiment involving rBGH is still ongoing. But other nations have refused to make guinea pigs of their own citizens. Canada, Australia, New Zealand, Japan, Israel and all European Union countries have banned rBGH and do not accept our treated dairy imports. The United Nations Food Safety Agency, representing 101 nations worldwide, unanimously ruled not to endorse rBGH milk. Today the United States is the only developed nation which allows humans to drink milk from cows given artificial growth hormones.

While the US continues to allow this dangerous drug trial, and while our tax dollars go to encouraging dairy consumption, our nation's milk-drinkers are putting themselves at risk for the development of a range of chronic diseases and ailments. Some of these may take decades to manifest. Others are already causing harm.

Cancer

Scientists don't argue about the fact that some cancers are hormone-dependent. They can't dispute the fact that the highest rates of hormone-dependent cancer, such as cancer of the breast, endometrium, ovary, prostate, testes and colon, are found in North America. They don't, however, agree about the role that our hormone-treated milk and our hormone-treated meat play in those realities.

Several studies in humans, animals, and cell cultures have shown that elevated levels of IGF-1 in humans stimulate the growth of breast, colorectal, prostate and other cancer cells.[91,92, 93] The exact nature of the link between IGF-1 blood levels and cancer remains unclear, but the association between circulating IGF-I level is strong enough to cast grave doubt on Monsanto's assurance that rBGH is perfectly safe.

One of the company's main assertions—that IGF-1 is destroyed in digestion—is patently false. While a sixty-second internet search will still produce multiple unsupported statements to this effect today, IGF-1 is _not_ destroyed by human digestion. Instead, IGF-1 is readily absorbed across the intestinal wall. Additional research has shown that it can be absorbed into the bloodstream where it can influence other hormones.[94]

Many scientists and health professionals believe that the US approval process for this drug was deeply flawed and that the cancer risk poses a serious public health threat. The Cancer Prevention Coalition, The Center for Food Safety, Consumer's Union, the American Public Health Association, American Nurses Association and many other organizations are still working toward an outright ban. The American Cancer Society (ACS) has no formal position regarding rBGH.

Early Puberty

Kids grow up fast these days. Entirely too fast, it seems. About 15 percent of American girls now begin puberty by the age of 7. One in 10 white girls begin developing breasts by that age, which is twice the rate seen in a 1997 study. Among black girls, 23 percent hit puberty by age 7.[95] Boys in the US are also showing signs of early puberty.

Maturing too early carries a whole set of psychological and social problems for the child, but since early puberty has been correlated with hormone-related cancers, there's even more cause for alarm. For decades there's been speculation that milk, which evolutionarily would have been limited to very young children, may be playing a role in this tide of early puberty.

Scientist have demonstrated that IGF-1 is key to the timing of puberty and that its administration triggers the onset of puberty in laboratory animals.[96] Data analyzed from the NHANES study published in 2012 showed cow's milk consumption associated with early menarche and height gain in adolescence. These researchers speculated that the signals sent by milk might have both immediate as well as longer-term impacts on the timing of sexual maturation.[97] Other research has also found earlier maturation related to milk consumption [98]

Some experts have suggested that this alarming rate of early puberty is attributable to obesity. There's no question that heavier girls experience puberty sooner. But rather than a *cause* of precocious puberty, obesity may well be another *effect* of the growth hormones and antibiotics that are used to make our food animals fat.

Others dismiss the association by claiming that girls today are drinking less milk than their mothers did. But since 1970, Americans have tripled individual cheese consumption, to nearly 33 pounds annually. Cheese, as well as butter, ice cream, yogurt, infant formula and thousands of other products and processed foods containing rBGH milk are sold in the US without labeling.

Few scientists are ruling out the impact of pollutants and endocrine disrupting chemicals in the environment. Our children now live in a virtual ocean of estrogenic chemicals. But again, pouring hormone-like chemicals on the morning's breakfast cereal would seem to add to the problem. Until large epidemiological studies are done to see whether or not early puberty in developing children is associated with eating growth hormone-treated foods, we can expect this massive feeding experiment to continue.

Acne

Many doctors, and certainly many parents, have long suspected a link between milk consumption and adolescent acne. A large body of research in the last decade has lent validity to that suspicion. Studies suggest that the association is caused not by fat, but by hormones and bioactive molecules present in cow's milk.

Researchers who examined the data from 47,355 women in the second Nurses' Health Study found that not only was the intake of milk during adolescence associated with a history of teenage acne, but that association was strongest with skim milk.[99] Years later the same research group conducted a prospective study on 6,094 adolescent girls and found that a greater consumption of milk was associated with a higher prevalence of acne and no association was found with milk fat.[100] Investigation into milk consumption and teenage boys yielded the same positive association between skim milk and acne.

After noting that acne can be regarded as an "indicator disease" of western nutrition, the researchers concluded that the "restriction of milk consumption or generation of less insulinotropic milk will have an enormous impact on the prevention of epidemic western diseases like obesity, diabetes mellitus, cancer, neurodegenerative diseases and acne."[101]

Allergies

The protein in cow's milk is the cause of one of the most common food allergens, especially in children. Life-threatening reactions are rare, but the symptoms can be quite unpleasant and may manifest in asthma, eczema (an itchy rash), rhinitis (inflamed nose), wheezing, vomiting, and mild to severe gastrointestinal distress. The most common way to test for food allergies is with an "elimination diet," in which all common allergy-causing foods are eliminated over a few weeks until symptoms lessen.

Lactose Intolerance

Lactose intolerance, also called lactase deficiency or *hypolactasia*, is the inability to metabolize lactose, the sugar found in milk which accounts for roughly half its calories. Symptoms of lactose intolerance include abdominal pain, bloating, flatulence, diarrhea, nausea and acid reflux.

While the condition is almost non-existent in infants, approximately 30 to 50 million American adults have some degree of lactose intolerance by age 20. The disorder affects some populations more than others. Seventy-five percent of all African-American, Jewish, Mexican-American, and Native American adults are lactose intolerant. Ninety percent of Asian-American adults are lactose intolerant. The condition is least common among people with a northern European heritage. [102]

According to the National Institute of Health (NIH), many people mistakenly believe that their symptoms are related to lactose intolerance without being properly diagnosed.[103] Some sensitivity may not mean that you have to give up all dairy. NIH data suggests that people with lactose malabsorption can tolerate 12 grams of lactose (equivalent to one cup of milk), particularly if eaten with other foods.

Parkinson's

Finally, several large cohort studies have suggested that high intakes of milk products may increase the risk of Parkinson's disease, the degenerative condition affecting movement and balance. [104, 105] Findings rule out both calcium and fat as responsible for the effects, but pesticides and other neurotoxic contaminants are still under suspicion. Because male milk drinkers were 2 to 3 times more likely to develop the condition, some researchers have also speculated that the cause may be the steroidal properties of Vitamin D, with which milk has been fortified since the 1930s.

The Raw Milk War

One of the food debates where opinions, and sometimes more than opinions, are clashing in a volatile way has been termed the "raw milk war," and in this case it's not just a figure of speech. Gun-carrying officers have raided organic dairy farms, seizing equipment and destroying dairy products. Private clubs and retail outlets for raw and unprocessed foods have been raided in California and in other states, and in some cases criminal offense charges have been filed. Authority for these armed raids comes from The Food Safety Modernization Act, which gives the FDA almost unlimited authority to decide if food is harmful.

At issue is *pasteurization*, the process named for French scientist Louis Pasteur, by which harmful microbes in perishable food products are destroyed with heat. USDA standards in the US require milk to be heated to 71.7 °C (161 °F) for 15 to 20 seconds. Pasteurization does not destroy all pathogens, but it kills many responsible for the transmission of a variety of deadly diseases. The process is credited with eliminating the scourges of typhoid and tuberculosis in the 1800's and many view it as one of the greatest of modern scientific breakthroughs.

The raw milk advocates, however, see things quite differently. For them, pasteurization has evolved into a great evil that threatens both public health and the environment. In creating a commodity dairy market, they believe that pasteurization has destroyed the dairy industry and family farms, and greatly contributes to deteriorating air and water quality, even as it forces cows to be fed soy protein concentrates, antibiotics and hormones. They argue that pasteurization substantially increases the IGF-1 levels in milk and destroys important vitamins and that raw milk consumption can prevent and treat allergies and asthma, lactose intolerance, even cancer.

Raw food advocates frame the debate as a freedom of food choice issue, calling the FDA out on hypocrisy both for continuously allowing known toxins into the food supply and allowing those who choose to harm their health in the consumption of too much sugar, artificial non-food-based items, alcohol, and cigarettes to do so freely. Proponents of unpasteurized milk insist that if milk is obtained from humanely raised cows that are grass fed and handled hygienically, then there is little problem with disease.

While there's not an abundance of research on the effects of pasteurization, a recent meta-analysis of forty studies found that the process exerts minimal effects on milk's nutritive value. Vitamins B12 and B3 decreased; vitamin A increased; concentrations of vitamin B6 were unchanged. The researchers found raw milk consumption was not associated with cancer (two studies) or lactose intolerance (one study), but six studies acknowledged that raw milk consumption may have a protective association with allergy development.[106]

Licenses for raw milk dairies have multiplied as the demand for what advocates describe as "real" milk over "dead" milk increases.

Doing a Body No Good

Even putting the issue of pasteurization aside, many experts now believe that the potential risks of milk-drinking far outweigh its benefits. Dr. Michael Klaper is one of them. Klaper, who grew up on a dairy farm, is now convinced that "the human body has no more need for cow's milk than it does for dog's milk, horse's milk, or giraffe's milk."[107] The nutritionists at the Harvard School of Public Health don't go quite that far, but they're also convinced that dairy is not part of a healthy diet. In the recent release of Harvard's "Healthy Eating Plate" food guide, dairy products were conspicuously absent. The Harvard experts thumbed their noses at the American Dairy Association and the USDA, declaring their guide to be based on sound nutrition research, not influenced by food industry lobbyists. [108]

Any debates, however, about the advisability of including milk in the healthy diet will have to address one indisputable fact. No non-human animals naturally drink milk beyond weaning; nor do any animals naturally drink the milk of other species.

Consumers Speaking Out

The milk front is one place in the **Great American Food Fight** where we're actually making progress. Consumers have voiced their demand for rBGH-free milk loudly and clearly, and the dairy sector is responding. Of the 100 top US dairy processors, 40 have declared themselves either partially or completely rBGH-free, including Kroger, Safeway Dairy Group, Anderson Erickson and Publix Super Markets, Sam's Club and Costco. Even Wal-Mart has announced that its private label Great Value milk will no longer come from treated cows. Retailers also are getting in on the trend. Starbucks went rBGH-free at the end of 2007, as did Chipotle Restaurants.

All of that consumer power is having an impact: A 2007 USDA survey found that just 17.2 percent of U.S. dairy cows are on genetically engineered growth hormone, down from 22.3 percent in 2002. The battle's not over, but it looks like free speech and the consumer's right to know may prevail.

Non Dairy Milks

Technically, milk can only be obtained from lactating animals and the dairy industries have legitimate objections to calling any plant-based product "milk." That being said, there are a variety of products which are similar in color and consistency to animal milks and which can serve as substitutes for people who are lactose intolerant or who have concerns about the safety of animal milk.

Almond Milk

Almond milk is now commercially available, but it can actually be made at home from finely ground toasted or raw almonds and water. It has a protein content similar to dairy milk, but without the lactose.

Except in those recipes that require a high fat content, it makes an excellent substitute for milk products in cooking.

Coconut Milk

Now that coconuts are emerging from the decades of bad publicity and erroneous information about saturated fat and cholesterol, many consumers are turning to coconut milk as a full substitute for dairy milk. Made from the squeezed extraction of coconut meat mixed with water, it has storage advantages over cow's milk, as well many health benefits not found in dairy. As noted in Chapter 5, the fatty acid found in coconut milk is lauric acid, which becomes monolaurin in your body. Monolaurin has antiviral, antibacterial, and antifungal properties. Coconut milk is available unsweetened and sweetened with cane sugar or sugar substitutes.

Rice Milk

Rice milk is another dairy-free beverage commonly used by those who are lactose-intolerant or those who wish to avoid consuming dairy products. It's made from boiled rice, rice syrup and rice starch. Some commercial brands, however, may contain polyunsaturated fats, sweeteners and emulsifiers, so read those labels carefully.

Soy Milk

A fuller discussion of soy as a genetically engineered food crop is taken up in Chapter 8, but it must be noted here that soy milk is perhaps the most popular substitute for dairy milk. A viable alternative to cow's milk for those with lactose intolerance, commercially fortified soy milk is also a good source of protein, iron, B vitamins and calcium, some evidence has suggested that consuming soy milk can have harmful side effects in certain circumstances.

Soy milk contains phytoestrogen, a hormone similar to estrogen. Phytoestrogens may have an effect on hormone-related cancers, particularly breast cancer and prostate cancer. Isoflavone, a type of protein found in soy, also raises concern. High isoflavone consumption has been linked to decreased fertility in animal studies and lowered sperm count in human males.

According to the American Thyroid Association, drinking soy milk may also interfere with your body's ability to absorb thyroid medication.

Dried and Powdered Milk

Dried milk is produced by forcing milk through small holes at high temperatures and extreme pressures. In the case of non-fat dried milk, it's skim milk. As with all over-processing, nutrients are destroyed, so some manufacturers may enrich or fortify the dried product with calcium, protein and other vitamins and minerals. The cholesterol also becomes oxidized, but in the case of skim milk, at least, the amount of damaged cholesterol is negligible.

Dried and powdered milks are suitable for long term emergency food storage, but beyond the reduction of fat and cholesterol—which are not the chief dangers of whole milk anyway—they offer few other advantages. Gluten intolerant consumers should read labels carefully, as some products may contain trace amounts of wheat.

Cultured Dairy Foods

Cultured dairy foods are made from milk which has been fermented with one of the strains of *Lactobacilli,* lactic acid bacteria, many of which are now grown in laboratories. The fermentation process increases the shelf-life of the product, as well as adds to the taste and improves the digestibility of milk. Fermented dairy products include buttermilk, sour cream, yogurt, and a wide range of cheeses.

Cheese

America is a nation of cheese-eaters. On average we consume over 30 pounds per person per year. If you're one of those cheese lovers, but have concerns about the growth hormones present in milk, you'll be more concerned about cheese, in which those hormones become concentrated. It can take 10 pounds of milk to make one pound of cheese.

The good news is that the hormone can be avoided. Small American processors have made hormone-free cheese for a decade, and now even the big names, like Kraft, are offering rBGH-free lines of cheeses. Most imported or European cheeses (goat or sheep or cow's milk cheese) will be made with no additional hormones Aged or hard cheeses, including cheddar, Gouda and Swiss, have little or no lactose.

Yogurt

Easily digested, easily absorbed, and rich in calcium, yogurt can be a healthful dairy food, assuming you know what you're buying. In theory, yogurt is made from culturing cream or milk with live enzymes and good bacteria, but here in the US, yogurt is one of those products for which the FDA has not defined a statement of identity. This omission allows lots of products to happily exploit yogurt's healthful reputation, without actually containing live and active cultures. Such products include yogurt-covered candies and pretzels, and yogurt-containing salad dressings. Many popular name-brand "yogurts" will contain live cultures, but may also contain dozens of other ingredients like sugar, fructose syrup, high fructose corn syrup, colorings, and other additives and fillers. Stick to plain, unflavored yogurts without added sweeteners, thickeners or preservatives. Many major yogurt manufacturers (Yoplait, Dannon, Nancy's All Natural) are now going hormone-free.

Butter

We've discussed butter as a spread and a solid cooking fat in Chapter 5 and argued there for choosing butter over margarine or spreads containing Trans fats.

To get butter minus the artificial hormones, antibiotics, and pesticides, you'll have to buy organic, but butter is one of the places where organic may be a bargain. Organic butter holds its shape better and the superior taste may also mean you'll use less of it.

Eggs

Eggs have fallen victim to the bad science and general confusion about cholesterol. In spite of the fact that we now know that dietary cholesterol is not the main culprit in coronary heart disease, and in spite of the fact that no research has ever linked egg consumption to heart disease, the myth persists, and a significant number of us still think eggs are off limits. Indeed, a survey conducted by the Egg Nutrition Center found that that nearly one out of four healthy adult Americans still avoids eggs for fear of dietary cholesterol. The bad press that eggs has received means that many of us are missing out on egg nutritional benefits.

Eggs contain 13 essential vitamins and minerals, high-quality protein, and important antioxidants. Egg yolks are an excellent source of choline, an essential nutrient that aids brain function in adults and contributes to fetal brain development and helps prevent birth defects. Research links two antioxidants found in egg yolks, lutein and zeaxanthin, to reduced risk for age-related macular degeneration (AMD), the leading cause of blindness in people over 50.

Choosing to put eggs back in our diets, however, won't necessarily make things simple for the consumer. There are still problems in knowing which type of eggs to choose as well as the ethical dilemmas surrounding egg production.

Organic vs. Non-organic Eggs

To be certified as organic, eggs must be produced from hens that have been fed certified-organic feed which was produced without synthetic pesticides or herbicides, antibiotics, or genetically-modified crops. No synthetic pesticides can be used to control external and internal parasites. Typically, organic eggs are also produced from hens in cage-free systems.

Organic eggs cost more because it costs the farmers more to give the chickens organic feed and requires more room to let them roam outside of cages. This cost can sometimes be significant, an average of about a dollar more per dozen eggs. For many consumers, that's a price worth paying, but the ethical issues surrounding battery-cage poultry production aren't simplified by organic egg production. Since male birds don't lay eggs, they are superfluous to organic egg production. In the words of United Poultry Concerns, "the baby brothers of all hens used for all egg production—regardless of the label—are suffocated to death in trash cans, electrocuted, gassed, or ground up alive as soon as they break out of their shells. For every "free-range," "cage-free," or "organic" hen, a baby rooster is born and trashed. No federal laws protect chickens from abuse under any label.[109]

Unfortunately, unless you know the farmer who raises them, the extra cost of "free range" or "cage free" labeled eggs may be going to clever marketers anyway. These terms are not regulated by the FDA or USDA and thus are essentially meaningless.

Animal Care Certified Eggs

If your egg-buying concerns also extend to animal welfare, you may want to know about the three certification programs for egg-laying hens verified through third-party auditing.

The **Certified Humane** label is a program of Humane Farm Animal Care. It means that egg-laying hens are raised uncaged, inside barns or warehouses. Hens are allowed to engage in natural activities and have sufficient space for nesting, perching, and dust-bathing, since stock density is regulated. No antibiotics or hormones are administered. Beak cutting is allowed under this standard.

American Humane Certified is a program of the American Humane Association. This label allows both cage confinement and cage-free systems, although animals may be confined in "furnished cages" not much larger than a legal-sized sheet of paper. Forced molting through starvation is prohibited, but beak cutting is allowed.

Animal Welfare Approved is a program of the Animal Welfare Institute which claims the highest animal welfare standards of any third-party auditing program. The birds are cage-free and continuous outdoor perching access is required. They must be able to perform natural behaviors such as nesting, perching and dust bathing and must be allowed to molt naturally. There are requirements for stocking density, perching, space and nesting boxes. Birds must be allowed to molt naturally. Beak cutting is prohibited.

Omega-3 Eggs

As egg sales have declined, driven by consumer perception that eggs are a high cholesterol food, the industry has responded with a "designer egg," re-engineered to calm cholesterol worries and to take up some of the slack in falling sales. Apparently it's working. These specialty eggs now account for 16% of US egg sales.

These alternative eggs are produced by feeding hens diets that are rich in Omega-3 fatty acids. This feed usually consists of high alpha-linolenic acid flax seed and fish oils, but may include other grains and seeds. The resulting egg has as much cholesterol as conventional eggs, but the new ratio of good vs. bad presumes that the eggs may reduce cholesterol levels. (*See Chapter 5, The Big Fat Lies About Fat.*)

While we were initially suspicious even of the efficacy of Omega-3 egg production, the peer-reviewed studies that we looked at do, indeed, confirm that these eggs can have three to six times the amount of Omega-3 fatty acids found in regular eggs. That still doesn't make egg choices easy.

These Omega-3 results, as one study stated, are "similar to those of egg yolks produced by free range hens feeding on green leafy vegetables, fresh and dried fruits, insects, worms, etc."[110] And it will still take an omelet of these re-engineered eggs to equal the Omega-3 found in a three ounce portion of salmon. Since Omega-3 eggs can be quite expensive, even pricier than free range eggs, health conscious buyers may want to opt for more ethically produced products. More cost-conscious consumers may simply choose to eat fewer eggs and acquire Omega-3 in other foods.

Brown vs. White

Brown eggs may be slightly more expensive than white ones because brown egg-laying breeds are often larger and thus more expensive to raise, but they are not more nutritious or "natural." Eggshell color depends completely on the breed of the hen. It's not related to quality, flavor, or nutritive value.

Processed Eggs, Egg Substitutes

Processed eggs, like liquid egg whites or dried egg whites, are actually egg shells broken by special machines, then pasteurized before being further processed and packaged into liquid, frozen or dried form. Some processed egg products may also contain preservatives and flavors or color additives.

Eating in the Meantime

- Cow's milk, when exposed to light, can lose significant amounts of vitamin A, riboflavin (a type of B vitamin), and vitamin D. Tests in which milk samples in translucent plastic jugs were exposed to dairy-case levels of light showed that more than 50 percent of some vitamins can be lost after just 15 hours. Milk in opaque paperboard cartons is not affected by light and thus retains its nutritional value longer.

- Sheep and goats are never injected with rBGH. It's also safe to buy imported European and Canadian cheeses and other dairy products, as rBGH is banned in these countries.

- A guide to hormone-free dairy can be found on The Great American Food Fight website. Remember also that all certified organic milk in the United States is rBGH-free.

- Labels reading "No bST" and "No rBGH" mean the same thing. No artificial bovine growth hormones.

- Unless you have a good physician-recommended reason for doing so, don't leave eggs out of your children's diet, or your own. You'll have to make your own decision about Certified Organic or Omega-3 eggs, but your only option for guaranteeing that eggs are produced under humane conditions is to buy them locally from a farmer you know.

- National chains like P.F. Chang's, Outback Steakhouse, Chili's and Rosa Mexicano now have menu items for the lactose intolerant.

- Giving up dairy doesn't mean that your diet has to be calcium-deficient. Many plants have as much calcium as milk. A Non-Dairy Calcium Chart appears in the Appendix..

Chapter 8. Genetically Modified Food

The major biotech players and the industry shills in their pockets are quick to accuse those who oppose the genetic modification of food crops of being "anti-science." We're the Luddites, we're told, not just standing in the way of progress, but morally equivalent to climate change deniers in obstructing the only possible path forward for feeding the world.

From the very beginning, however, there was pitiful little science in the rush to push GMO foods down the public throat. In 1992, when the FDA formally issued its presumption that GE foods were GRAS, it was well aware that not only were they not recognized as safe, but that no consensus as to their safety existed in the scientific community at large. The FDA had suppressed the objections of its own experts who argued that the processes of genetic engineering and traditional breeding were different and thus entailed different risks.[111] The official policy declared the opposite, claiming that the FDA knew nothing of significant differences, and since GMO foods were substantially equivalent there was no need to label them. This process would be repeated in other countries which looked to the US regulatory system as a sanctioning entity for the approval of transgenic crops.

With the science on genetic engineering officially established, at least by Monsanto and the FDA, there was no need to reassess the safety of new commercialized GE crops. Public funding for conventional breeding all but dried up as resources poured into new GE research and development. Over the next decades, the corporatization of the world's food supply would get underway in earnest, with a handful of biotech transnationals buying up the key segments that control the American food chain. As of 2013 Monsanto, Syngenta, DuPont, Dow, Bayer and BASF controlled 75 percent of private sector plant breeding research, 60 percent of the commercial seed market, and 76 percent of global pesticide sales. [112]

The biotech industry hasn't made it easy to add to the science on GMO safety. Estimates made by scientists themselves suggest that 95% of those researching in the area of genetic engineering are funded by industry. Only 1% of our own USDA biotech research funding goes to any type of GMO risk assessment. Independent researchers have difficulty accessing the materials for GM biosafety research because Monsanto, who owns the patents, won't supply the seeds, and has strict licensing agreements that prevent independent examination of their products. Scientists whose work has resulted in negative findings for transgenics have been severely punished, their research suppressed by leading editorial decisions by peer-reviewed journals, and in some cases their careers destroyed. [113, 114, 115]

Now, many years into humanity's largest feeding experiment, the safety of GE crops for human consumption has still not been adequately assured. There still have been no mandatory human clinical trials of genetically engineered crops, no tests for carcinogenicity or harm to fetuses, no requirement for long-term testing on either humans or animals, and limited testing for allergenicity. There have been no epidemiological studies of the possible effects of the consumption of GE crops on human health.

Despite the lack of objective investigation into these critical areas, there are many who think that the GMO debate is over. Confident that the rising rates of chronic diseases seen in this country have nothing to do with GM food, industry spokespeople, journalists, politicians, and food "experts" make sweeping, unequivocal claims about the safety of GM technology and consider the science settled. The truth is very different.

No Scientific Consensus

A stunning illustration of just how far we are from genuine scientific agreement came on October 21, 2013, when the European Network of Scientists (ENSSER) issued a statement disputing the contention that there is a consensus on the safety of GM foods. The statement was compelled, according to the group,

> . . . because the claimed consensus on GMO safety does not exist. The claim that it does exist is misleading and misrepresents the currently available scientific evidence and the broad diversity of opinion among scientists on this issue. Moreover, the claim encourages a climate of complacency that could lead to a lack of regulatory and scientific rigour and appropriate caution, potentially endangering the health of humans, animals, and the environment.[116]

The scientists, physicians and legal experts who initially signed the group statement provided seven reasons for the need to issue the statement.

To wit:

1. There is no consensus on GM food safety
2. There are no epidemiological studies investigating potential effects of GM food consumption on human health
3. Claims that scientific and governmental bodies endorse GMO safety are exaggerated or inaccurate
4. EU research project does not provide reliable evidence of GM food safety
5. List of several hundred studies does not show GM food safety
6. There is no consensus on the environmental risks of GM crops
7. International agreements show widespread recognition of risks posed by GM foods and crops.

The original list of 90 signatories has now grown to over 300, with ENSSER calling for further independent scientific inquiry and informed public discussion on GM product safety.

Promises Unfulfilled

Given the obstacles to the kind of independent, non-industry funded scientific inquiry that ENSSER advocates, it appears that we'll have to wait a little longer for knowledge of the true human health costs of genetically modified agriculture. As for many of the other pledges made by Big Biotech in the rush to commercialize GM crops, the science is already coming in. Here's what we're learning about the false promises and technological failures of genetically engineered food.

GM Crops Will Increase Yields

The main tenet justifying GMO technology since the mid-90s has been that GMO crops would produce higher yields and thus aid in combating world hunger in the face of overpopulation and climate change. The "GMO's will feed the world" meme has been the cornerstone of biotech public relations campaigns for almost twenty years now—time enough, one might think, to see ample evidence of this most hopeful of promises coming to fruition.

In 2009, however, the Union of Concerned Scientists became the first to substantially deflate this particular hot air balloon. The UCS report, entitled Failure to Yield, found that "despite 20 years of research and 13 years of commercialization, genetic engineering has failed to significantly increase U.S. crop yields."[117]

More recent reports have arrived at the same conclusion. University of Canterbury researchers in New Zealand compared data on agricultural productivity in North America with Western Europe over the last 50 years. The team found that the biotechnologies used in North American, specifically the use of GM seeds, are actually lowering yields and increasing pesticide use as compared to Western

Europe. Instead, the researchers found "that the combination of non-GM seed and management practices used by Western Europe is increasing corn yields faster than the use of the GM-led packages chosen by the US. [118]

In a USDA-funded study published in February 2013, University of Wisconsin scientists looking at 20 years' worth of data from test plots found that several types of GMO seeds (including Monsanto's Roundup Ready varieties) were also producing a lower yield than conventional seeds. Only one seed—a corn that produces its own pesticide to combat the corn borer — offered any significant yield benefit.[119] In other words, planting most genetically modified seeds results in less harvest per acre than planting non-genetically modified seeds.

It seems that American farmers may actually be getting, in some cases, more of certain crops produced per unit of land over a specified amount of time. But the increased yield is mainly due to traditional breeding or improvements in agricultural practices. There is no good evidence that GM technology increases crop yield.

GMO Crops Will Require Fewer Pesticides

In the mid-1990s agribusinesses began advertising GM seeds that promised to reduce a farmer's use of toxic pesticides. The benefit to the environment as well as to the farmer made this particular promise especially appealing and encouraged the adoption of Roundup ready seed. Unfortunately, the "fewer pesticides" promise may be the most tragic misrepresentation of all for farmers and consumers.

Research is showing that GE crops are only more productive during the first few years, after which they consistently need increased applications of herbicides/pesticides. Since GMO crops were introduced 1996, U.S. farmers have used 404 million more pounds of pesticide than they would have with just conventional crops.

In the next chapter, *Produce and Poisons*, you'll find a discussion of the specific human health dangers of pesticides, but suffice it to say that reducing pesticides has definitely not been one of the benefits of GMO technology.

GM Crops Are Better for the Environment

Another of the benefits promised by the biotech industry was that GM crops would be more sustainable over the long term, lessening the drain on natural resources, particularly water. Monsanto, for example, continues to claim itself a "sustainable agriculture company", empowering farmers "to produce more from their land while conserving more of our world's natural resources such as water and energy." But if the concept of sustainability means anything at all to the rest of us, Monsanto's green wash is also hogwash.

Water

Water is becoming an increasingly scarce resource as global water pollution reaches epic proportions. Here at home, 40% of our rivers and 46% of our lakes are already too polluted for fishing, swimming, or aquatic life. Two-thirds of our estuaries and bays are either moderately or severely degraded from nitrogen and phosphorus pollution.[120] While there are many causes of water pollution, genetically modified crops are playing a significant role in worsening the water crisis. They contaminate fresh water and ground water supplies and are less water-efficient than conventional crops.

Two studies from the US Geological Survey (USGS) have found that Monsanto's Glyphosate, known by its trade name Roundup, is commonly found in rain and rivers in agricultural areas in the Mississippi River watershed. It's now a common component of the air and rain in the Midwest during the spring and summer.

Agricultural use of glyphosate increased from less than 11,000 tons in 1992 to more than 88,000 tons in 2007, and yet, as Paul Capel, USGS chemist and an author on this study admits, "we know very little about its long term effects to the environment." [121]

We do know, however, that GM seeds don't just need more fertilizer and pesticides than conventional crops, they need more water, too. Even Monsanto's DroughtGard corn, engineered from the cspB gene and the only product specifically developed to be drought resistant, hasn't delivered on its promise of "getting more crop per drop." A recent USDA analysis, using Monsanto's own data, shows that DroughtGard produces only modest results, and only under moderate drought conditions. The report estimates that *cspB* corn would increase the overall productivity of the U.S. corn crop by only about one percent. That's the same rate that classical breeding techniques and improved farming practices have increased drought tolerance in U.S. corn over the past several decades. And DroughtGard does not improve water use efficiency.[122]

Biodiversity

As a new, alien, and invasive species, GMOs pose a unique threat to biodiversity. Their impact can be readily seen in the emergence of super weeds and super insects, but the toxins produced by genetically engineered crops also threaten biodiversity by destroying beneficial insect species (lacewings, ladybugs, moths, butterflies, bees, etc.), and by hastening the disappearance of a wide range of native plant species.

Since the 1900s, some 75 percent of plant genetic diversity has been lost as farmers worldwide have abandoned their multiple local varieties for genetically engineered seeds. Three-quarters of the world's food is now generated from only 12 plants and five animal species.[123] The implications of this loss for human health, indeed, for human survival are profound. We depend on these varieties for food, medicine, livelihood, purification of our water, and stabilization of our climate.

It may take some time to comprehend the large scale losses to biodiversity from the Bt toxin and the flood of glysophate entering the planet's ecosystems, but the death march of GM agriculture through contamination of native and organic crops is clearly observable and measurable right now.

For more than a decade GMO proponents, with the backing of the USDA, insisted that genetic contamination could never happen. But it does. And with frightening speed and efficiency. Genetically modified pollen is spread naturally on the wind, carried by insects, animals, and humans and has already become a serious threat to native species as well as to the livelihoods of non-GE and organic farmers.

In September 2000, StarLink, a variety of Bt corn unapproved for human consumption was discovered in taco shells in the United States. In 2009 a federal jury awarded 2 million US dollars to two Missouri farmers after their rice crop was contaminated with an experimental variety of rice that the company had been testing since 2006. Its developer, Bayer, admitted that despite "best practices" it has been unable to control the spread of its genetically-engineered organisms. In 2013 Oregon wheat was found to be contaminated by a variety of GE seeds developed by Monsanto.

Most of the soybean supply in the U.S. is already contaminated with genetically modified seeds. In Canada, non-GMO canola is now virtually nonexistent. Mexico's indigenous corn varieties have been contaminated by GM corn. Organic maize production in Spain is dropping as the acreage of GM maize production increases from cross-pollination with GM maize. In Hawaii, GM pollen drift has contaminated organic papaya to the point that most growers have given up. The story is being repeated, across the globe, and with a multitude of crops.

Contamination of non-GM and organic crops has already resulted in massive financial losses by the food and feed industry, involving product recalls, lawsuits, and lost markets is already in the billions of dollars. The cost to our planet's biodiversity is incalculable.

Soil

GM crops are almost universally found in monocultures—large areas of land devoted to a single crop or species. Monocultures deplete soil of valuable nutrients. Crops grown decades ago were much richer in vitamins and minerals than the varieties most of us get today. While post-war industrial agriculture in general has been the culprit, both in soil depletion and the disappearance of topsoil, the cultivation of GE crops is likely making a bad situation much worse.

The latest science suggests that genetically engineered plant cultivation can seriously disrupt soil ecology by reducing microbial diversity and decreasing soil fertility over time. Studies have demonstrated that Monsanto's BT toxin, which was claimed to kill only harmful insects, persists in decomposing plant parts and in the soil, impeding soil flora recovery and impacting plant health and growth in subsequent growing seasons. [124]

The mechanisms for this are just beginning to be understood, but there is certainly no evidence to suggest that introducing genetically engineered organisms into the soil is going to address problems of global food scarcity. On the contrary, at the rate that GE plants may be reducing soil fertility, the consequences could well be global famine.

There is no criterion by which the cultivation of GM crops can be judged as better for the environment. The evidence shows they've been an environmental nightmare.

GM Will Keep Food Prices Low

You would expect one of the benefits of GM technology to be reduced cost for farmers and therefore ultimately for the consumer. In fact, GMOs have not lowered prices at all. In comparison with conventional crop seeds, GM seeds are significantly more expensive. But that's not the worst of it. As conventional growers make the switch to genetically modified varieties they become locked into a monopolistic system which requires the constant repurchase of seed as well as the acquisition of a variety of other company products like fertilizers and pesticides.

> Worldwide, GM crops are not lifting small farmers out of poverty, because these smallholders can't afford the cycle of sterile seeds and patented fertilizers and pesticides.

We've seen what can happen to prices in seed monopolies in examples like India. In a decade, Monsanto gained control of 95 percent of the cotton seed market, and seed prices jumped 8,000 percent. Vandana Shiva, physicist, environmental activist and longtime critic of industrial agriculture, has pointed to cases in which small farmers in India have killed themselves when the debt they've taken on to buy seed, fertilizer, and pesticides became too crushing. Monsanto has tried to delink the epidemic of farmers' suicides in India from the company's growing control over the cotton seed supply, but nearly 300,000 Indian farmers have committed suicide since 1995 after being driven into insurmountable debt. [125]

In the US food prices have also risen with escalating seed prices since the introduction of genetically modified varieties. Worldwide, GM crops are not lifting small farmers out of poverty, because these smallholders can't afford the cycle of sterile seeds and patented fertilizers and pesticides. Rather they exacerbate poverty by undermining the sustainable agricultural systems that farmers have developed over millennia and creating dependence on the products produced by a few US corporations. GM crops are designed to save big farmers time and money only if they are involved in large-scale, high-tech agriculture.

The simple logic behind food prices was outlined by Sarah Gilbert in an article for *Daily Finance*. "In a roundabout way," says Gilbert,

> "the widespread use of genetically modified seeds whose prices are controlled by a single company must increase the cost of food. Farmers are prohibited from saving their own seed and are beholden to the company for its pesticide; soil bereft of both helpful and beneficial organisms requires far more fertilizer; the production and transportation of the fertilizer and pesticide and seeds require fossil fuels. Far more external, annual inputs are required in a genetically engineered agricultural system. With the increased use of energy, demand is greater, oil prices go up, climate change is exacerbated, everything gets more expensive." [126]

The truth of the matter is that most of the benefits of GMOs accrue to biotech firms and large farmers, leaving little to balance out the risk to consumer health or to our environment. There is no good evidence that currently grown GM crops have had a positive impact on global food prices.

When all global agriculture is centralized in the hands of a few unelected individuals, who do you imagine will be in the catbird seat in terms of food prices?

> There is no good evidence that currently grown GM crops have had a positive impact on global food prices.

GMOs Will Solve Food Scarcity

As we've already seen, GMO agriculture does not significantly increase crop yields. But the argument that GMOs will feed the world becomes more ludicrous when we realize that, in fact, most GM crops are not grown to produce food for people at all. They are being grown to provide animal feed, bio fuels, in the form of bio-diesel and bio-ethanol, and cotton. The production of biofuels in particular has diverted millions of acres of land away from food production, spurred speculation in grains which has driven up prices, and driven 30 to 75 million into hunger.[127]

GMO proponents, however, insist that exploding population growth and food scarcity means that GMOS are essential for meeting global food demand by 2050. This is pure biotech propaganda resting on completely false notions. Starvation and malnutrition are not functions of population or of relative food scarcity.

Let's dispense with the easy one first. The one about exploding world population growth. Despite the sensationalist doomsday prophecies, the rate of global population growth has actually slowed. And it's expected to keep slowing. Already, more than half the world's population is reproducing at below the replacement rate. Indeed, according to experts' best estimates, the total population of Earth will stop growing within the lifespan of people alive today. [128]

A shrinking, or even stabilizing rate of population growth will still leave us with a great many mouths to feed. So, what about food scarcity? Like runaway population growth, food scarcity is also a myth.

> GM seeds, most of which aren't even planted for food, don't even address the real causes of hunger.

We already produce more calories (over 3,500) per day per person on the planet than we actually need. (Studies suggest that most of us don't need more than about 2,000). That means that today we're already producing nearly twice the food necessary for everyone on the planet to be adequately fed. Additionally, there's the matter of food waste. Estimates suggest that from 30 to 50% of our food simply gets thrown away.

As Greenpeace has noted, most hungry people live in countries that have food surpluses rather than deficits. Here in the US, where there is no food scarcity, one in six people live in hunger. Hunger is not about food supply and population. It's about access and distribution to food, and the economic, social, and political factors that foster poverty.

Genetically modified food is not "required" to meet the demands of overpopulation. GM seeds, most of which aren't even planted for food, don't even address the real causes of hunger. As we've seen, future food security for all of us is under threat from climate change, our diminishing natural resources, and planetary loss of biodiversity. But GM technology is not providing solutions to those problems. We'll have to find another way to feed tomorrow's world.

A Better Way

Globally, a series of recent reports are pointing to a much more viable path for feeding the world. They reveal that non-GMO, low input, sustainable farming practices can alleviate hunger, reduce dependency on fossil fuels and chemicals, use resources efficiently, and create healthier communities.

The Rodale Institute's Farming Systems Trial is America's longest-running side-by-side comparison of organic versus conventional farming. Begun in 1981, the study compared a conventional farm using recommended fertilizer and pesticide applications with an organic animal-based farm and an organic legume-based farm. The two organic systems received no chemical fertilizers or pesticides.

After an initial decline in the first years of the study, over time the organic systems produced higher yields, especially under drought conditions. Corn and soybean yields were the same across the three systems. The organic approaches, however, used an average of 30 percent less fossil energy, conserving more water in the soil, induce less erosion, maintain soil quality and conserve more biological resources than conventional farming does. [129]

In developing countries, too, study after study shows that organic and agroecological techniques—farming methods that combine scientific understanding about how places work (their ecology), with farmers' understanding of how to make their landscapes useful to humans (agriculture) can provide much more food per acre than conventional chemical-based agriculture. Field studies show that the yield increases from shifting to organic farming are highest and most consistent in exactly those poor, dry, remote areas where hunger is most severe.

A fair number of agribusiness executives, international agricultural experts and ecological scientists believe that a large-scale shift to organic farming would not only increase the world's food supply, but might be the only way to eradicate hunger. [130]

A Global Awakening

The case against GMOs has gained strength in the last few years as real science and the real experiences of farmers have exposed the dangers of GE organisms and the emptiness of Big Biotech's promises. A few years ago, there were only sixteen countries that had total or partial bans on GMOs. Today there are at least sixty four counties with significant restrictions or outright bans on GMOs. In the European Union, mandatory labeling, in effect since 1997, has all but driven genetically engineered foods and crops off the market. The only significant remaining GMOs in Europe today are imported grains (corn, soy, canola, cotton seed) primarily from the U.S., Canada, Brazil, and Argentina The tide may be turning as more governments institute total or partial bans on GMO cultivation, importation, and field-testing.

In October 2013 a Mexican judge ruled that, effective immediately, no genetically engineered corn can be planted in that country. This means that companies like Monsanto will no longer be allowed to plant or sell their corn within the country's borders.

At about the same time, the County Council for the island of Kauai passed a law that mandates farms to disclose pesticide use and the presence of genetically modified crops. The bill also requires a 500-foot buffer zone near medical facilities, schools, homes and other locations.

In the South American fight, Peru has become the lead country after approving a 10-year ban on importation, production and use of GMO foods in the country. The ban is aimed at protecting Peru's ever increasing exports of organic and native food products and to safeguard the country's rich variety of native plant species from cross pollination with genetically modified crops. Ecuador, Kenya, and Russia, Japan, Australia and New Zealand have also instituted bans on growing GMO crops. More and more of the world's educated consumers are pushing for outright bans or at least GMO labeling.

The U.S. Battle for Labeling

Food manufacturers make GMO-free products for consumers in 64 other countries for one of two reasons: Either because consumers in those countries have demanded that GMOs be banned from their food supplies, or because consumers have demanded GMO labeling laws. Here in the US we may be a long way from getting an outright ban on

GMOs, but we're steadily moving closer to the labeling laws that, according to surveys, up to 93% of us now want.[131]

Although labeling bills were narrowly defeated in California and 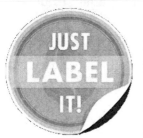 Washington, the fight definitely didn't end there. To date, more than 70 bills have been introduced in over 30 states to require either GE labeling or prohibition of genetically engineered foods.

On April 16, 2014, in a huge victory for transparent food labeling, the Vermont Senate passed H.112 by a vote of 28-2, following up on the passage of a similar bill in the Vermont House last year. The legislation requires all GMO foods sold in Vermont to be labeled by July 1, 2016. As expected, the Grocery Manufacturers Association, whose 300-plus members include giants like Monsanto, Dow, Coca-Cola and General Mills, have sued the state of Vermont, but at long last the Right-to-Know Movement has real momentum and overwhelming grassroots pressure can deliver a real victory.

While GM labeling is slowly gaining ground, the Non-GMO, GM-Free, and Organic labels are taking US health food markets by storm. The Non-GMO Project is a non-profit organization offering America's only third party verification and labeling for non-GMO food and produce. 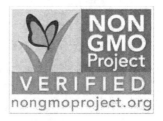 The organization's Non-GMO Project Verified seal only first appeared on products in 2010, but it has since become one of the fastest growing labels in the natural products industry. While American consumers wait for government to mandate labeling, we're seeking out these private labels for assurance that the food we buy is not manufactured with GE ingredients.

What's in the Pipeline

According to the Biotechnology Industry Organization, many new GM crops are scheduled to reach the market within the next six years.

Among these are Roundup Ready versions of alfalfa, lettuce, tomato, Bt apples, GE bananas, sunflowers, and herbicide resistant varieties of rice and strawberries. Genetically engineered salmon has already received FDA approval. Other GE fish, such as tilapia, trout and flounder are also in the pipeline.

The number of genetically engineered crops lining up in the FDA pipeline emphasizes the need for transparent labeling. Consumers deserve a choice.

What's at Stake

Even if you're part of that slim 7% sliver of consumers who don't know much, or care much, about GMO labeling, you ought to care, and deeply, about the latest attempts to make the food you're eating none of your business. A bill recently introduced in Congress would have nullified all state efforts, like Vermont's, to label GMO foods. It aimed to effectively decide the issue, permanently, for all American consumers.

The legislation championed by Rep. Mike Pompeo (R-Kan.) and dubbed by opponents *the Deny Americans the Right to Know* Act or DARK Act, would block state GMO labeling laws and codify the broken *voluntary* GMO labeling system. It would have allowed new GMO traits to be used in food regardless of whether FDA had even completed a review and specifically prohibited Congress or individual states from requiring mandatory labeling of GMO foods or ingredients. HR 4432 also aimed to legalize the use of the word "natural" on products that contain GMOs.

There was a lot at stake in this audacious, insulting, anti-American, bill. Fortunately, after passing the House, the DARK act was blocked in the US Senate in March of 2016. We still don't have GMO labeling, but for now consumers have staved off another advance of the food corporatocracy. If we don't want another whole series of food choices taken from us, we need to continue to fight.

Eating in the Meantime

While we continue to fight for the right to know what we're eating, many consumers would like to avoid eating GMOs as much as possible. It takes effort and vigilance to eliminate genetically modified food from your diet, but there are steps you can take to minimize risks for you and your family and to cast your own ballot for non-GMO farming and Right to Know Labeling.

Know Which Foods Are Likely GM.

Right now very few fruits and vegetables are genetically modified. Currently about half of Hawaiian Papaya is GM and only a small amount of Zucchini and Yellow Squash are GM. The main GM sources are the crop plants, corn, soybeans, canola, cottonseed, and sugar beets. Unfortunately, these crops appear in a multitude of products and derivatives.

Additives – There are many enzymes, artificial flavorings, and processing agents that are produced by GM bacteria, yeast or fungi. To avoid them, either buy organic or stick to non-processed foods.

Honey – Some Canadian honey comes from bees collecting nectar from GM canola plants. This has shut down exports of Canadian honey to Europe.

Sweeteners containing aspartame – A building block of aspartame, the amino acid phenylalanine is usually manufactured with the aid of genetically modified E. coli bacteria. It is commonly found in chewing gum and diet beverages. *See Chapter 10.*

Vegetable Oils – Most generic vegetable oils and margarines used in restaurants and in processed foods in North America are made from soy, corn, canola, or cottonseed. Unless these oils specifically say "Non-GMO" or "Organic," they are probably genetically modified.

Understand Organic Labels.

In the United States, federal legislation defines three levels of organic foods. Products made entirely with certified organic ingredients and methods can be labeled "**100% organic**," while only products with at least 95% organic ingredients may be labeled "**organic**."

Your best assurance that your food plants that have not been genetically modified or that animals have not been fed genetically modified feed is the 100% organic seal.

The USDA Organic label may appear on products that contain at least 95–99% organic ingredients (by weight). The remaining ingredients are not available organically but have been approved by the National Organic Program.

Products with less than 70% organic ingredients will not bear the USDA Organic seal.

Warning: The "natural" label, or any variant of it, **is not a substitute for the Organic label**. Many natural foods contain ingredients that have been grown with pesticides or are genetically modified. This applies to eggs, as well. Eggs labeled "free-range," "natural," or "cage-free" are not necessarily GMO-free. Look for eggs labeled 100% organic.

Whenever possible, look for "Non-GMO Project" verified labels or symbols or labels that specifically state "Made without genetically modified ingredients."

Read those Produce Label Stickers.

When buying produce, look at the PLU # (price look up) sticker affixed to the item. Remember that a 5-digit number beginning with an 8 indicates a GM food. A 5-digit number beginning with a 9 indicates organically grown produce.

Purchase 100% Grass-fed Beef.

Most cattle in the U.S. is raised as grass-fed, but spends the last portion of its life in feedlots where it may be given GM corn to increase intramuscular fat and marbling. If you're trying to stay away from GMOs, make sure the cattle were 100% grass-fed or pasture-fed (sometimes referred to as grass-finished or pasture-finished).

This advice also applies to meat from other herbivores like sheep. There is a slight possibility that the animals were fed GM alfalfa, although this is less likely if you buy meat locally. With non-ruminants like pigs and poultry that cannot be 100% grass-fed, it's better to look for meat that is 100% organic.

Shop Locally.

Although more than half of all GM foods are produced in the US, most of that comes from large, industrial farms. By shopping at farmers' markets, food cooperatives, and community supported agriculture programs (CSAs), we strengthen our own local and regional food systems, put more money in the hands of farmers, and eat more safely.

Chapter 9. Produce and Poisons

As every farmer or gardener knows, if you plant it, they will come. Those creepers, crawlers and diseases that like our crops as much as we do are always lurking, and the battle to control them is as old as agriculture itself. Ancient Romans controlled weeds with salt. The Chinese applied sulfur to control mold and bacteria as early as 1000 BC, and also pioneered other minerals, like arsenic, as both insecticide and herbicide. The extracts from plants and trees—tobacco leaves, chrysanthemums, the strychnine tree—have been used throughout recorded history to control rodents, insects, and disease.

Versions of many of these more or less "natural" pesticides are still in use today, but now, as then, they are difficult to purify and hard to produce in large quantities. The real breakthrough in pest control had to wait for the development of synthetic chemistry. It came, in a big way, in 1939, when Swiss scientist Paul Hermann Müller discovered the insecticidal properties of the synthetic chlorinated hydrocarbon we know as DDT.

The discovery of DDT represented a revolutionary advance in the battle against bugs. The chemical was not only cheap to make and easy to apply, but it had some other pretty amazing properties, described by terms that are familiar now to most anyone who's ever owned a lawn. DDT was broad spectrum, meaning it was toxic to a wide range of insect pests. It was nearly insoluble in water, so it didn't get washed off by rains, and it was persistent in the environment, meaning it didn't break down rapidly and didn't have to be reapplied often.

Those qualities, as we now know, are exactly the ones that make pesticides so dangerous to humans and to the environment, too, but back then DDT was being hailed as a miracle. The chemical was used widely to treat crops, but also for non-agricultural purposes. It was used to delouse soldiers in WWII, to combat malaria in tropical regions, and to keep down mosquitos here at home, too. "Mosquito trucks" patrolling neighborhood streets and fogging DDT into summer evenings were once an American commonplace. Müller was awarded the Nobel Prize for his discovery in 1948.

Yet even during those halcyon days for DDT, there were some scientists beginning to worry about its effects. Early research in the 1950s found that DDT and its derivatives accumulated in human and animal fat tissue. It showed up in human breast milk at remarkably high concentrations, and compared with healthy controls, the serum of patients dying of cancer revealed significantly more of the DDT derivative, DDE.

Others were concerned about the effects of DDT on the environment. Because DDT was so long-lasting—it's one of the contaminants we now call POPs, for Persistent Organic Pollutants, it was being taken up in the air and soil by non-target organisms and transported long distances in water by marine animals and fish.

In 1962, marine biologist and naturalist Rachel Carson not only gave voice to those concerns, but essentially launched the modern environmental movement with the publication of her best-selling work, *Silent Spring*. The book documented the detrimental effects of pesticides on animal life, particularly on birds, in which the pesticide load became concentrated as they ate contaminated aquatic plants, plankton, and fish. DDT and its relatives altered the calcium metabolism of birds in a way that resulted in eggshells so thin they were unable to support the weight of incubating birds. Breeding failures resulted in the decimation of the Brown Pelican populations in much of North America, in extermination of the Peregrine Falcon in the eastern United States and southeastern Canada, and in declines in populations of Golden and Bald Eagles, White Pelicans, and others. Carson also predicted the ability of pest species to evolve a resistance to pesticides.

Carson's work provoked a massive backlash from the chemical industry, but it also elicited an enormous public outcry, prompting President John F. Kennedy to appoint a Science Advisory Committee to review the issue. The Committee's investigations ultimately led to the canceling of DDT registration for agricultural use in 1972.

The ban on DDT, however, did not in any way curtail enthusiasm for producing new synthetic chemicals for agricultural use. Today, more than two billion pounds of pesticides are used each year in the United States to control weeds, insects and other organisms. More than 17,000 pesticide products are currently on the market.

The Pesticide Treadmill

The validity of Rachel Carson's prediction that targeted insects and weeds would evolve their own resistance to synthetic pesticides has been demonstrated for more than half a century. Massive outdoor spraying of DDT in third world countries subject to malaria was already being abandoned in the 1970s, not because of government bans, but because DDT had lost its ability to kill the mosquitoes. In the decades since, as insect larvae, rodents and weeds developed poison resistance to the latest new pesticide within a few scant generations (*their* generations, not ours), farmers have found themselves caught on a "pesticide treadmill," forced to use more and more, and increasingly toxic, chemicals.

One justification for the marked increased in pesticide and herbicide use that we've experienced in recent decades is the same one we hear for the necessity for genetic engineering. We've got to feed the world! The truth, however, is that this ever-increasing toxic deluge has not materially reduced crop losses for US farmers. While we're using more pesticides than at any time in human history, we're only holding our own, or in some cases, actually losing ground in the battle with pests and weeds.

Insects, plant pathogens, and weeds now reduce US crop production by about 37% per year. That's a loss rate, according to Dr.

Patricia Muir, of Oregon State's Department of Botany and Plant Pathology, "that is essentially **unchanged since the dawn of the chemical age!**" (Emphasis hers). In essence," says Muir, "we are using ever greater quantities of pesticides to achieve a fairly constant level of control."[132]

In some cases, losses to pests have actually increased: For example, in the US, between 1945 and 1989 losses to insects increased 2-fold (doubled: up from 7% loss to the current 13%) in spite of a 10-fold increase in both the amount and the toxicity of the insecticides being used.

> Over 98% of sprayed insecticides and 95% of herbicides reach a destination other than their target species

Losses to weeds in US agriculture have decreased slightly since 1942 (to 1989); from about 14% loss to about 12%. However, during this time there was about a vast increase in herbicide use.

As we saw in Chapter 8, the development of GE crops, designed in some cases to contain their own pesticides, has not resulted in the reduction of pesticide use. On the contrary, genetic engineering is only serving to keep us on the pesticide treadmill.

The environmental impact of all that poison is often much greater than what is intended by those who use them. Over 98% of sprayed insecticides and 95% of herbicides reach a destination other than their target species, with long lasting consequences.[133] One of those non-target species is human.

Pesticide-Induced Diseases

Links to pesticide exposure have been found in numerous studies that evaluate the causes of many preventable diseases. These include asthma, autism and learning disabilities, birth defects and reproductive dysfunction, diabetes, Parkinson's and Alzheimer's diseases, and several types of cancer.

ADHD, Learning Disabilities

Researchers at the Harvard School of Public Health studied 1,139 children ages 8 to 15, about 10% of whom had ADHD. All of the children submitted a urine specimen for testing. The urine of children with ADHD had significantly higher levels of byproducts of organophosphates, the class of pesticides to which DDT belongs. The higher the level of these byproducts in the urine, the greater the chance the child had ADHD. Those children who had any pesticide level in their urine were twice as likely to have learning disorders as children with no detectable pesticide levels. Especially troubling is the fact that this was not a high exposure sample of kids living on farm or near pesticide manufacturing plants. These kids were exposed to normal levels of pesticides.[134]

Autism

Autism rates have simply skyrocketed in the last decade. In the period between 1997 and 2008, autism prevalence among boys increased 261%. Prevalence among girls increased more than 385% over the same period. [135]

Mounting evidence suggests gestational pesticides exposures are strong candidates for the development of autistic spectrum disorders.[136] In California's rich Central Valley agricultural region, a 600% increased incidence in autism was observed among children up to 5 years of age for births from 1990 to 2001, yet only one-third of the rise could be explained by identified factors such as changing diagnostic criteria for autism or a younger age at diagnosis. [137]

The National Academy of Sciences now estimates that about one third of all neurobehavioral disorders, like autism and ADHD, are caused either directly by pesticides and other chemicals or by interaction between environmental exposures and genetics.[138]

Birth/Fetal Effects

Even the EPA acknowledges that laboratory studies have shown that pesticides cause birth defects. While its effects on humans remains unclear, glysophate in particular has been associated with deformities in a host of laboratory animals. One French study done in 2005 found that Roundup and glyphosate caused the death of human placental cells.[139] Another study, conducted in 2009, found that Roundup caused total cell death in human umbilical, embryonic and placental cells within 24 hours.[140] Few follow-up studies have been undertaken.

A review of recent studies on birth and fetal effects can be found under Information Services on the Beyond Pesticides.org website.

Cancer

The associations between many types of cancer and occupational or environmental exposure to pesticides are so extensive that they would fill many books. Fewer studies, however, have addressed dietary exposure. That's changing. And the news is not good.

Researchers from the University of California Davis recently looked at dietary exposure in children and adults for eleven foodborne toxins for which the EPA has established cancer "benchmarks." These benchmarks are the exposure levels that would generate one excess cancer per million people over a 70-year lifetime. Among the toxins included were the pesticides, or pesticide by-products arsenic, dioxin, dieldrin, chlordane, and DDE.

Arsenic pesticides are still legal in the United States. Dioxins are by-products of herbicide and pesticide production. Dieldrin is an insecticide, now banned in most of the world. Chlordane is a banned pesticide, and DDE, of course, is that breakdown product of DDT.

The study found that, while adults exceeded the cancer benchmark for many of these toxins, the margin of exposure was much greater for children. All of the participating children (100%), exceeded the cancer benchmark levels. In fact, children exceeded the cancer benchmark levels 10-fold for DDE, nearly 100-fold for dieldrin, and over 100-fold for arsenic and dioxins. Preschool-age children had significantly higher estimated intakes of 6 of the 11 compounds compared to school-age children.[141]

Research has established that even low doses of glyphosate can induce human breast cancer cell growth. The estrogenic activity may be compounded in the presence of some naturally occurring properties of food crops. Glyphosate-based herbicides are widely used for soybean cultivation, for example. Studies have found an additive estrogenic effect between Glyphosate and genistein, a phytoestrogen in soybeans.[142]

Parkinson's

Parkinson's is a degenerative disease of the central nervous system which affects millions worldwide. In yet another example of the tragic correspondence between disease rates and pesticide use, Parkinson's is also on the rise. In 2010 (the last year for which data is available), there was 4.6% increase in the number of deaths attributed to this disease.

The motor symptoms of Parkinson's disease result from the death of dopamine-generating cells in the brain. While the exact cause of Parkinson's is unknown, the clearest evidence is for an increased risk of PD in people exposed to certain pesticides.

Numerous studies have implicated the pesticides paraquat, rotenone, lindane, and dieldrin in the development of Parkinson's disease due to their ability to kill dopaminergic neurons. It appears that glyphosate may have similar capabilities. [143, 144]

Reproductive Dysfunction

Because hormones themselves act at extremely low levels, biological processes controlled by hormones are extraordinarily sensitive. This means there often is no "threshold" or "safe" dose for endocrine disrupting compounds that exist in many pesticides. It's not surprising that they have been implicated in a range of reproductive disorders. Pesticides have been tied to early puberty, to decreased semen quality, as well as issues with menstruation, ovulation and fertility in women.[145]

Obesity and Diabetes

Accumulating evidence from in vitro, in vivo, and epidemiological studies are also linking human pesticide exposure with obesity, metabolic syndrome, and Type 2 diabetes. [146, 147]

In a study conducted by the Mercer University School of Medicine to examine whether pesticide exposure played a role in worldwide childhood obesity, researchers observed nearly 6,800 subjects aged 6 to 19. Individual exposure to environmental pesticides was determined through the use of urine tests, identifying the concentrations of pesticide residues. The researchers found a higher prevalence of obesity in the participants with high urinary concentrations of a pesticide known as 2,5-dichlorophenol (2,5-DCP), one of the most widely used pesticides on the globe.

The growing list of chemicals suspected of contributing to obesity in humans also includes persistent organic pollutants like polychlorinated biphenyls (PCBs) as well as DDT and its breakdown product, DDE. Some studies suggest that even prenatal exposure may be associated with overweight in children. [148]

The Pesticide-Induced Diseases Database, launched by Beyond Pesticides, provides access to epidemiologic and laboratory studies based on real world pesticide exposure scenarios. Look for the link to the database under **Information Services** at the *BeyondPesticides.org* website or in our **Pesticides** Battle section at *TheGreatAmericanFoodFight.com*.

Kids and Pesticides

Pesticides are dangerous for all of us, but children are especially vulnerable. They metabolize faster, taking in more food, water and air than adults, but are less able to process contaminants. Prenatal and early childhood exposure to neurotoxic pesticides during critical development windows can lead to lifelong effects. Even very low levels of exposure can derail development, undermining the ability to learn and resulting in significant drops in IQ. Yet, despite what we know about the special vulnerabilities of children, there is no corner of the planet where pesticides are not impacting our children's health.

As pesticide use has increased over the past thirty years, so have the rates of childhood cancers, birth defects, early puberty, asthma, diabetes, obesity, developmental disorders and learning disabilities. The majority of studies have focused on environmental or industrial exposure but children consume pesticides in food and water also.

While it remains the best source of nutrition for infants, decades of breast milk sampling shows that all over the globe nature's perfect food has been contaminated by pesticides. Low levels of pesticide residues, including eight known to be toxic to the nervous system, five that disrupt hormones, and eight that are potential carcinogens have been found in baby food.[138] In samplings of produce commonly eaten by school-age children, USDA residue testing has found metabolites of dozens of different pesticides.[138] The herbicide, atrazine, is found in 94% of US drinking water tested by the USDA.

We've known for some time that children, because they are still developing, are more vulnerable to pesticide exposure than adults and that diet delivers the bulk of that exposure. We now know how to offer our children at least some protection. Research has convincingly demonstrated that organic diets can significantly lower children's exposure to pesticides. [149]

Pesticides and Wildlife

A new class of systemic, neurotoxic pesticides that are known to be particularly toxic to honey bees has rapidly taken over the global insecticide market since their introduction in the 1990s. This new class of insecticides, the neonicotinoids, act in the central nervous system of insects, resulting in paralysis and death. Neonicotinic residues can accumulate in pollen and nectar of treated plants and represent a potential risk to pollinators.

The website for Beyond Pesticides (Beyondpesticides.org) also has a comprehensive directory of companies and organizations that sell organic seeds and plants. Included in this directory are seeds for vegetables, flowers, and herbs, as well as live plants and seedlings.

Regulating Pesticides

Since 1972 the primary authority for registering and regulating pesticides has rested with the Environmental Protection Agency (EPA). By law, in order for a company to register and sell a pesticide, it is supposed to be subject to a rigorous review process which includes a period for public comment, analysis of scientific studies, and evaluations by the agency's in-house science experts. This process in itself is reactionary rather than precautionary because EPA officials rely on research data submitted by pesticide manufacturers and the burden of proving that a chemical is harmful rests on the public. Yet even the scant safeguards that the law requires are systematically ignored. Pesticide manufacturers do everything they can to drag out reviews of their products, often for decades. Lawsuits are pending to force the EPA to follow the law and speed up review, but thousands of pesticides enter the market without safety testing or public awareness.

The EPA also continues to assess the risk of each pesticide individually, failing to consider cumulative and synergistic effects. The US Geological Survey has not only found pesticides in every water source it tested, but multiple types of toxins.

A better, common sense precautionary approach to protecting us would assess alternatives to highly hazardous pesticides rather than accepting public exposure to pesticides as a necessary evil. Such a shift will require fundamental federal policy reform.

Although the EPA is also required by law to consult with the U.S. Fish and Wildlife Service on pesticide registration, it has failed to complete a single consultation in the last ten years despite repeated formal requests from the wildlife agency and the unambiguous requirements of the Endangered Species Act.

Eating Pesticides

We need to be concerned about pesticide residues in fruits and vegetables, but not so concerned that we stop eating these healthiest of foods. The established benefits of lowering heart disease and cancer are far greater than the risks. We can mitigate risks, however, and save a little money, too, by knowing which foods are the most hazardous for pesticide contamination and which ones are relatively "clean."

The Dirty Dozen and Clean Fifteen

By now most consumers have heard of the "Dirty Dozen" and "Clean Fifteen" lists offered by The Environmental Working Group. These are annual comprehensive lists outlining the 12 most pesticide-contaminated fruits and veggies, and the 15 produce options that are the least contaminated. The 12 most contaminated are peaches, apples, sweet bell peppers, celery, nectarines, strawberries, cherries, pears, imported grapes, spinach, lettuce and tomatoes. The least pesticide residue is found on onions, avocado, sweet Corn (Frozen), pineapples, mango, asparagus, sweet peas (frozen), kiwi fruit, bananas, cabbage, broccoli, papaya.

When it comes to those on the dirty dozen list, it's best to cough up the extra dough and get organic. With the clean fifteen, it's up to the individual consumer to decide if organic is worth the extra protection.

Is Organic Worth the Price?

According to a survey by the Harvard School of Public Health, half of the country's adults say they buy organic food often or sometimes. Since organics usually cost more, those of us paying the price are doing so for a variety of reasons. Lots of us are convinced that, as a general rule, organically grown food just tastes better. Some of us are concerned about genetic engineering and the environmental impact of large-scale conventional farming. A few studies are beginning to find that organic fruits and vegetables average higher nutrient levels. But the decision to pay more is also about what we're *not* getting. In the case of pesticides, we're not getting a lot.

Organic food production is subject to many more regulations aimed to protect ecological and human health than conventional agriculture. The regulation of pesticide may be the area of starkest contrast. In conventional agriculture, synthetic pesticides with known health effects may still be registered for use. Even the EPA concedes that its pesticide registration process is no guarantee of safety and it specifically prohibits manufacturers from making claims like "safe," "harmless," or "non-toxic to humans and pets," even with accompanying phrases like "when used as directed." Additional "inert" ingredients in the formulations are not taken into consideration in the registration process, even though many of these inert ingredients are known toxins themselves. Under the organic regulations, only naturally derived pesticides and a very few low-toxicity synthetic ingredients, like boric acid, are permitted. Inert ingredients in these products must be approved for organic production.

Most organic farmers depend on non-chemical solutions for crop protection. Pests and diseases are controlled by focusing on healthy plants and good soil, by rotating crops, and employing biological controls such as beneficial insects. Instead of herbicides, organic farmers rely on good crop rotation, cover cropping, mechanical cultivation and mulching to limit weeds. No-till organic agriculture is a new approach that combines some of these practices at once.

The issue of pesticide residue on organic produce has been surprisingly controversial. Because some organic crops have tested positive for synthetic chemicals, and because "green" labeled foods have been found to contain significant residue levels, it's not difficult to find commentary on the internet claiming that organic foods are as pesticide-laden as conventionally grown crops. There is now good data from three independent sources to prove otherwise.

The Pesticide Data Program of the U.S. Department of Agriculture; the Marketplace Surveillance Program of the California Department of Pesticide Regulation; and private tests conducted by Consumers Union have compared residue data on 20 crops. All three data sets showed striking, highly statistically significant differences. The analysis showed convincingly that organically grown foods have fewer and generally lower pesticide residues than conventionally grown foods. This pattern was consistent across all three independent data sets. Organic foods typically contain pesticide residues only one-third as often as conventionally grown foods do. Highly statistically significant differences were also found in the frequency of multiple residues, with conventionally grown produce often containing residues of more than one pesticide, and in some cases up to 14 different chemicals.

Is Organic Food Pesticide Free?

Does that mean that organic food will always be pesticide free? No, it doesn't. Even the most conscientious organic farmers may still encounter situations that result in their crops testing positive for some level of pesticide residue. The spray "drift" from pesticide application, especially aerial ones, can reach organic farms, as well as our own backyards or our children's playgrounds. Another type of drift, volatilization drift, happens when a pesticide is applied to a field and then hours or even days later, the pesticide vaporizes from the surface of plants or out of the soil, creating an invisible vapor cloud that moves offsite. There's also the lingering, or legacy effects of DDT. Though DDT has not been used in the US for nearly 30 years, the pesticide and its breakdown products are still detected at low levels in a wide variety of foods eaten by Americans. Residues of DDT and DDE are still found in the soil of fields and forests treated years ago, and in the sediment of lakes and rivers. Crops grown in contaminated soil can still come in contact with these residues.

There is enough data now to say with certainty that organic food has significantly less pesticide content and is safer than conventional.[150] While the USDA claims that the amount of pesticide residue on conventional food is negligible, a study by the University of Washington showed that parents who feed their kids organic food significantly lower the amount of pesticide residue in their kids' bodies. In fact, an analysis of the children's urine showed they were exposed to six to nine times fewer toxic pesticides than those who ate a conventional diet.[151]

Judgment as to whether or not organic foods taste better may be subjective. But the judgment as to whether they're safer is not. Our household food choices can help not only to protect our own families, but to support and grow the market for foods produced without dangerous pesticides. Supporting organic agriculture helps all families live less toxically.

Eating to the Nines

Those annoying little stickers that must be peeled away from fresh fruits and vegetables are not meant for consumer education. They are PLU (price look-up) codes developed by the International Federation for Produce Standards to enable scanning and pricing of loose produce at the register. They can, however, provide information on how the food is grown if you know what to look for. .All **4**-digit number codes indicate that the food is conventionally produced, with all the chemical fertilizers, fungicides, and herbicides typical to cultivation of that crop. A 5-digit number beginning with an **8**, indicates a GM food. A **5**-digit number beginning with a **9**, indicates organically grown produce.

Unfortunately, since PLU labeling is optional, some GM foods may not have a PLU identifying them as such, but you can trust the **9**'s.

Eating in the Meantime

- Eating a variety of fresh produce reduces your exposure to any one contaminant.

- Although some organic food may test positive for trace residues of pesticides as a result of the background exposure in soil, air and water, organic foods are much less likely to have residues, and when found residue levels are well below those found and legally permitted in conventional food.

- Pesticide Action Network (PAN) maintains a searchable database for toxicity and regulatory information about pesticides at http://www.pesticideinfo.org/. PAN's What's On My Food? Database shows which pesticides are found on what foods, and cross-references this data with toxicological profiling. More pesticide resources can be found on our website at Greatamericanfoodfight.com.

- Per pound of body weight, babies consume about 60 times more fruits and vegetables than adults. This fact, combined with undeveloped digestive and immune systems, puts young children at the greatest health risk for pesticide residues. To minimize the effects, you might consider buying organic for those foods that your youngest children eat regularly.

- Washing conventionally grown fruits and vegetables helps a little to reduce the amount of pesticides they contain, but it won't eliminate them. Don't turn to soap to scrub off those pesky pesticides. Experts recommend using plenty of fresh, drinkable water and a vegetable brush to reduce pesticides as well as bacteria.

- When thinking about organic produce for your own family's consumption, think also about organic pest control for your own home, garden, and lawn. There are safe and effective alternatives to most of the harmful pesticides registered for use by the EPA.

- Beyond Pesticides.org has a comprehensive directory of companies and organizations that sell organic seeds and plants. Included in this directory are seeds for vegetables, flowers, and herbs, as well as live plants and seedlings.

- Remember that pesticides, by their very nature, are designed to kill living organisms. Avoiding them as much as possible is always the smart move.

Chapter 10. The Sour Truth about Sugar and Artificial Sweeteners

It won't come as a surprise to most readers to learn that Americans consume a lot of sugar. What may be shocking to many, however, is the true extent of sugar's toxicity. Sugar is by far the most ubiquitous and possibly the most dangerous and addictive food additive in the modern food supply. It's at the linchpin center of our diet-induced health crisis.

Too Much of a Sweet Thing

We've been growing our national sweet tooth fairly steadily since Christopher Columbus brought sugar cane to the new world. In 1700, the average person consumed about 4 pounds of sugar per year. By 1800, the average person consumed about 18 pounds per year. By 1900, the individual consumption rate had risen to 90 pounds of sugar per year.

In the mid twentieth century, however, developments conspired to make us really crave the sweet stuff. There was, of course, a general explosion in the manufacture and marketing of processed foods. And, as you will recall from Chapter 5, American consumers also became subject to national recommendations on reducing total and saturated fats. The food industry responded by increasingly substituting sugar, fructose, and high fructose corn syrup. By 1999, each American was consuming an average of 158 pounds of caloric sweeteners per year, the equivalent of about 50 teaspoons per day.

Obesity researcher and neurobiologist Dr. Stephen Guyenet has plotted the trend for sugar consumption in grams from 1822 to 2005. As you can see, it's a remarkably steep line – a trend so pronounced, says Guyenet, that should it continue, by 2606 the US diet would be 100 percent sugar. [152]

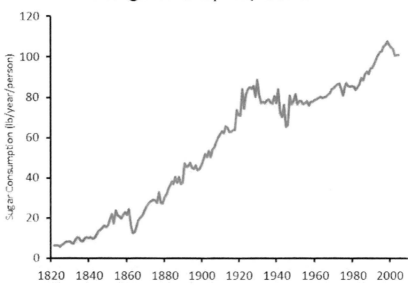

Average daily American consumption of added sweeteners has decreased slightly, down from the peak in 1999, but Guyenet's chart provides a stark illustration of how radically the American diet has changed in a short time. That change corresponds to an equally stark rise in many diseases.

Sugar and Disease

The most direct link between sugar and disease is to obesity which also links sugar to the host of obesity-related diseases including diabetes, hypertension, metabolic syndrome, cardiovascular disease, atherosclerosis, thyroid dysfunction, sleep apnea, reproductive disorders and more. While this book takes up other obesogenic factors in our industrialized food supply—the role of antibiotics, for example, as discussed in Chapter 6— it's difficult to exaggerate the role of sugar in weight gain and obesity.

The role that sugar plays in simply adding calories to the American diet is not widely disputed, but for decades the conventional wisdom has been that weight gain occurs when the "calories in, calories out" balance goes awry. If we take in more calories than we burn, regardless of whether those calories come from buttered yeast rolls or chocolate bon-bons, we're going to put on weight. If we persist in this imbalance, we'll become obese and thus vulnerable to the obesity-related risk factors for other diseases also.

That conventional wisdom has been challenged in recent years. It's not that simple, many experts are now telling us. That "calories in, calories out" equation is a gross oversimplification. The metabolic consequences of different calories are quite different and sugars specifically, rather than calories in general, are the real culprits in the obesity epidemic.

Insulin Resistance

All carbohydrates cause blood sugar (glucose) to rise, but sugars, often called simple carbohydrates, are most quickly converted to glucose. Think of them as dry kindling for a fast, hot-burning fire. When sugar is consumed in large quantities it drives up the secretion of insulin which, as we know, controls the levels of glucose in the blood. When insulin regulation fails to work properly, allowing blood sugar levels to rise too high, one result is the development of Type 2 diabetes, the chronic condition of excess blood glucose—a condition that effects 25.8 million children and adults in the United States alone.

Not even the American Diabetes Association is willing to say that over-consuming sugar "causes" diabetes, but the sugar/diabetes connections prove stronger with each passing year. Type 2 diabetes is not only on the rise in the US but in 175 other countries around the world—those countries where sugar availability in the diet is greatest.

Research shows that for every additional 150 calories of sugar (the amount in a 12-ounce can of soda) available per person per day, the incidence of Type 2 diabetes rises by 1%. [153]

While we've known for some time that being overweight or obese can predispose us to diabetes and other diseases, we haven't been eager to assign any disproportionate share of the blame to sugar. Americans are lazy and slothful we're told. We eat too much of everything, especially saturated fats, and we just don't get enough exercise. Sugar, say some, is merely a convenient whipping boy for our bad habits and national character.

That argument, however, is becoming harder and harder to sell as we advance our understanding of the biologic process of weight gain. The first breakthrough came in 1994 when Dr. Jeffrey Friedman and his research team at Rockefeller University discovered that the fat cells of genetically obese mice failed to produce a chemical called leptin. This previously unknown hormone serves as a master regulator of appetite.

Leptin Resistance

Leptin was the first *adipokine*, the first hormone shown to be made exclusively by fat cells. Also modulated by insulin, Leptin is often called the *satiety hormone*, because it turns off your appetite and can cause you to burn more calories. With continuous overexposure to the hormone, however, the leptin signaling stops working so well. Like learning to ignore the little boy who cried "wolf" too often, the brain stops responding to the leptin that the body is producing and doesn't tell us that we're full now and can stop eating. This condition, called leptin resistance, makes losing weight difficult, if not impossible. It's the reason that advice to eat less and exercise more can be all but worthless. It helps to explain what the obesity epidemic and the diabetes epidemic have proven so intractable.

It's the Sugar. *Really.*

This unfolding knowledge of how insulin and leptin talk to each other, and how leptin resistance works to shut down our satiety signaling, has convinced many that it's not the calories that are making us obese, it's the sugar. One of the nation's most well-known obesity experts, Dr. Robert Lustig, is among them. Lustig, a pediatric endocrinologist at the University of California at San Francisco, is waging a campaign to convince consumers, and other doctors, that sugar is the biggest perpetrator of our current health crisis. He's the author *of Fat Chance: Beating the Odds Against Sugar, Processed Foods, Obesity and Disease*, and creator of the YouTube video, "Sugar: The Bitter Truth" which has been viewed over three million times.

Lustig's message is that calorie for calorie, sugar makes us fatter than other foods. He argues that sugars are toxins, pure and simple, but its unique biochemistry makes fructose especially toxic and thus the main villain in the obesity epidemic.

While sucrose and fructose have the same caloric value, they are processed very differently by the body. Glucose can be metabolized by any cell in the body, where, assuming our signaling systems are working properly, insulin will direct it to energy use now or to fat storage for use later. Fructose, however, is metabolized almost entirely by the liver. There it doesn't trigger the release of the leptin hormone to tell us we're full or satisfied, so we keep eating. The fructose, especially around our midsections, is converted into triglycerides, or fat, and insulin resistance, metabolic syndrome, Type 2 diabetes, and obesity are the inevitable result.

Lustig has co-authored a report with the American Heart Association recommending that women consume no more than 100 calories of added sugars a day and men no more than 150, but US dietary guidelines provide no limit at all for added sugar. Other experts, like Dr. Mark Hyman, believe that our outdated dietary guidelines are causing us real harm. "As it turns out, "says Hyman, "sugar calories are deadly calories. Sugar causes heart attacks, obesity, Type 2 diabetes, cancer and dementia, and is the leading cause of liver failure in America." [154]

It's becoming clearer that sugar calories are much more dangerous than other calories. And, to make a bitter truth even more unpalatable, a growing body of recent research is showing that sugar is as addictive as hard drugs in programming our brains for physiological cravings.

Sugar Addiction

The evidence that sugar can be a substance of abuse and lead to a natural form of addiction had been accumulating for more than a decade before a Princeton team found the final incriminating piece in the cycle of craving, withdrawal and relapse that characterizes addiction. Researchers had already been able to induce sugar dependency in rats and even to demonstrate that sugar surpasses cocaine as a form of a reward. [155] But the Princeton team, led by Dr. Bart Hoebel, found that sugar-binging caused long-lasting changes to the brain and even increased the inclination to take on other drugs, like alcohol. After one month on a high sugar diet, the brains of the rats had adapted to higher levels of dopamine and had a reduced level of dopamine receptors. [156]

The research likening sugar to addictive drugs is definitely accumulating. Eric Stice, a neuroscientist at the Oregon Research Institute has used fMRI scans to show that sugar activates the same brain regions that are activated when a person consumes drugs like cocaine. [157, 158] Dr. Nora Volkow, Director of the National Institute on Drug Abuse, has done similar research using brain imaging techniques to show similarities between the brains of people who are obese and people who abuse drugs and alcohol. And very recent studies have observed the common biological basis for obesity and nicotine addiction.

It appears that the neural mechanisms that underlie obesity and drug addiction are so startlingly similar because to our bodies some foods, especially sugar, actually *are* drugs. And this drug is the most widely available in modern human society. That's a reality, as Dr. Volkow has noted, that makes the phrase "Just Say No!" sound like magical thinking.

Knowing Our Sugars

Discovering that we may have a sugar dependency doesn't necessarily doom us to lifelong obesity. But sugar is ubiquitous in our modern food supply and unlike cocaine, alcohol or nicotine, it's harder to identify and harder to avoid. The first step in fighting back is always closing the knowledge gap. In this case that means understanding the types of sugars, knowing how they behave in our bodies, and learning to identify and root out the source of hidden sugars.

Nutritive Sweeteners

Nutritive sweeteners are those that are naturally found in food. They include sucrose, which is in table sugar; fructose found in fruit and table sugar; galactose found in milk, and the sugar alcohols, that group of carbohydrate compounds that are not true sugars but are common sweeteners which contain calories and have some effect on blood sugar.

Sucrose

Sucrose is what we commonly call table sugar. It's a complex carbohydrate, or disaccharide, made from the combination of the two simple sugars, sucrose and fructose. When the body breaks down the complex carbohydrate sucrose, it absorbs the glucose and metabolizes the fructose, which can then be stored in the body. Sucrose occurs naturally in sugar cane, sugar beets, the sap of the sugar maple, in dates and honey. It's produced commercially from sugar cane or sugar beets.

Fructose

All plants produce sugar as a byproduct of photosynthesis. In fruits and vegetables that sugar is in the form of fructose, as readily available in canned apple juice as it is in a fresh apple, but with important metabolic differences. The effects of the fructose consumed directly from fruits and vegetables is mitigated by their fiber, which slows the rate of digestion, reducing the insulin response, leading to more stable blood sugar levels, and triggering satiety much quicker. The effects of a high sugar diet are compounded by the absence of fiber in the highly processed foods and fast foods that most Americans eat. It's all but impossible to over-consume fructose from fresh fruit and vegetable sources.

High-Fructose Corn Syrup

The most commonly added sweetener in processed foods and beverages is High Fructose Corn Syrup, or HFCS. It does not occur in nature but is manufactured through an enzymatic process that converts corn starch first into glucose and then into fructose. Its popularity as a sweetener in processed foods rests on several desirable characteristics. HFCS is as sweet as table sugar, it blends well with other foods, and helps foods to maintain a longer shelf life. Most importantly, thanks to government corn subsidies, it's much cheaper to use than sugar.

The United States leads the way in high fructose corn syrup consumption with a staggering average of 55 pounds per person per year. Our leadership in HFCS consumption and in global obesity and diabetes rates are inextricably connected, and again, it's not just the added calories that these sweetened process foods provide, but the specific nature of HFCS itself.

In another study undertaken by the same Princeton research team, rats with access to high-fructose corn syrup gained significantly more weight than those with access to table sugar, *even when their overall calorie intake was the same.* Rats fed high-fructose corn syrup also had more abdominal fat and elevated levels of triglycerides, two symptoms associated with obesity.

For Professor Bart Hoebel, who led the Princeton team, these findings dispute the claim that high-fructose corn syrup is no different from other sweeteners when it comes to weight gain and obesity. "Our results make it clear that this just isn't true, at least under the conditions of our tests," says Hoebel. "When rats are drinking high-fructose corn syrup at levels well below those in soda pop, they're becoming obese -- every single one, across the board. Even when rats are fed a high-fat diet, you don't see this; they don't all gain extra weight."[159]

Sugar Alcohols

Sugar alcohols, or polyols, are ingredients used as sweeteners and bulking agents. They're a natural ingredient in food and come from plant products such as fruits and berries. As a sugar substitute, they provide about a half to one-third fewer calories than regular sugar. They're converted to glucose more slowly, require little or no insulin to be metabolized, and don't cause sudden spikes in blood sugar. Because sugar alcohols are not completed absorbed by the body, however, high intakes of foods containing some sugar alcohols can lead to laxative effects, including abdominal gas, bloating and diarrhea.

The sugar alcohols commonly used in food products are sorbitol, mannitol, and xylitol. Sorbitol is on the GRAS list, while mannitol and xylitol are regulated as additives. The FDA has filed GRAS affirmation petitions for isomalt, lactitol, maltitol, HSH, and erythritol.

Non-Nutritive Sweeteners

Non-nutritive sweeteners, or artificial sweeteners, are synthetically derived sugar substitutes which provide little or no nutritional value. They are sweeter than natural sugars and are low calorie, but provide no energy and contain no vitamins and minerals. The FDA has given the GRAS status to six of these: Aspartame, Acesulfame-K, Neotame, Rebaudioside A, Saccharin, and Sucralose. A seventh, Cyclamate, was banned in the U.S. in 1970, but is currently under review for re-approval.

Aspartame

Aspartame, marketed under such brand names as NutraSweet, Equal and NatraTaste, is a synthetic derivative made up of a combination of the amino acids aspartic acid and phenylalanine. Free methanol is created from aspartame when it is heated to above 86 Fahrenheit (30 Centigrade). Methanol breaks down into formic acid and formaldehyde in the body, and formaldehyde, as we know, is a deadly neurotoxin.

Since its approval in 1989, aspartame has been the subject of considerable controversy, but the answer to the question, "Is aspartame safe for human consumption?" depends very much on who you ask. The industry, of course, asserts that aspartame is safe, but where independent analysis of peer-reviewed studies of aspartame have been undertaken, the conclusions are much different.

Dr. Ralph G. Walton of The Center for Behavioral Medicine analyzed 164 studies which were felt to have relevance to human safety questions. Of those studies, 74 studies had aspartame industry-related sponsorship and 90 were funded without any industry money. Of the 90 non-industry-sponsored studies, 83 (92%) identified one or more problems with aspartame. Of the 74 aspartame industry-sponsored studies, all 74 (100%) claimed that no problems were found with aspartame.

Some of the health concerns arising out of aspartame research include headaches, formaldehyde accumulation in the body,[160] fibromyalgia symptoms, depression, memory loss, diabetes risk, lymphoma-related illness [161] and weight gain.

Finally, for those who have the genetic metabolic disorder phenylketonuria (PKU), the amino acid, phenylalanine, which is an ingredient in Aspartame, poses a serious health concern. In individuals who have PKU, phenylalanine can cause mental retardation, brain damage, seizures and other problems. Federal regulations require that any food product that contains aspartame bear a warning stating: *Phenylketonurics: Contains phenylalanine.*

Currently, aspartame can be found in more than 4,000 products, some of which include gum, yogurt, diet soft drinks, fruit-juices, puddings, cereals, and powdered beverage mixes.

Acesulfame K

Acesulfame potassium, or Acesulfame K, or Ace K is a favorite sweetener of beverage companies and can be found in most diet sodas. Marketed under the names of Sunett and Sweet One, it is 200 times sweeter than table sugar but often blended with other sweeteners (usually sucralose or aspartame) to mask a bitter aftertaste. It cannot be metabolized by the body, and thus is a no calorie sweetener, but it does stimulate insulin secretion and susceptibility to cravings for sweetness.

While Acesulfame K has been an approved sweetener since 1988, its critics are far from satisfied that its safety has been assured. The FDA's approval was based on two short-term tests on rats and one on mice submitted by Hoechst, the manufacturer of the chemical. In 1996 the CSPI urged the FDA to require better testing before permitting acesulfame-K in soft drinks, but the FDA has still not required that these tests be undertaken. There have been few clinical trials on humans to date, but lab testing on animals have shown some problems including tumors to the lungs.

Some studies have shown that Acesulfame K can be ingested by the prenatal or postnatal mice through their mother's amniotic fluid or breast milk, and continue to influence sweet preference into adulthood.[162]

Acesulfame K contains methylene chloride, a known carcinogen. Long-term exposure to methylene chloride can cause headaches, depression, nausea, mental confusion, liver and kidney problems, visual difficulties, and cancer.

Saccharin

Saccharin, the oldest artificial sweetener, known as Sweet and Low, Sweet Twin, Sweet 'N Low, and Necta Sweet, is 200 to 700 times sweeter than table sugar but it has a bitter aftertaste.

Saccharin was first investigated as a health risk by the USDA in 1907 when Theodore Roosevelt was in office. Many studies have ensued since then, many of them linking Saccharin to cancer. In 1977 the FDA considered banning it when studies suggested it caused bladder tumors in male rats.[163] At the time, however, saccharin was the only artificial sweetener available. Public pressure prevailed on Congress to override the ban. The sweetener was allowed, provided it carried the following warning: "Use of this product may be hazardous to your health. This product contains saccharin which has been determined to cause cancer in laboratory animals."

In 2000, the National Toxicology Program (NTP) concluded that saccharin should be removed from the list of potential carcinogens, but the safety concerns of consuming products with saccharin remain even with the removal of the warning. In 1997 the CSPI responded to the request for removing saccharin from the list of potential carcinogens by stating that if saccharin is even a weak carcinogen, the unnecessary additives would pose a risk to the public.

Another possible danger of saccharin is reaction by individuals allergic to the sulfonamides in saccharin. Reactions include headaches, breathing difficulties, skin eruptions, and diarrhea. Many health groups also believe that the use of saccharin should be limited in infants, children, and pregnant women.

Sucralose

Aspartame's long-held position as the leading artificial sweetener has recently been supplanted by sucralose, marketed under the brand name *Splenda*. It's 600 times sweeter than table sugar, and contains no calories. It's rapidly become one of the most popular and highly consumed artificial sweeteners and can currently be found in over 4,500 products.

The FDA reviewed studies in human beings and animals and determined that sucralose did not pose carcinogenic, reproductive, or neurological risk to human beings. In 1998, it was approved for limited use, and in 1999, it was approved as a general-purpose sweetener.

Early research suggested that sucralose, for the most part, passed through the body without being metabolized. Recent studies, however, dispute this, showing that ingestion of sucralose can alter the amount and quality of the beneficial microbes in our gastrointestinal tract, may raise insulin levels and blood sugar, and can interfere with a wide range of prescription medications.[164]

Another serious safety concern arises from the formation of highly toxic chlorinated compounds, including dioxins, when Splenda is used in baking.[165] Beyond the obvious dangers of direct human consumption of these toxins, sucralose apparently does not break down in the environment. It survives water treatment plant purification techniques and is accumulating in our drinking water.

Symptoms that have been known to be associated with sucralose are gastrointestinal problems such as bloating, gas, diarrhea, and nausea, and skin irritations such as rashes, hives, redness, itching, and swelling. Additional symptoms are wheezing, cough, runny nose, chest pains, palpitations, anxiety, anger, moods swings, depression, and itchy eyes.

Splenda uses the antioxidant banner and an enticing picture of strawberries, raspberries, blackberries and blueberries to create the impression of being natural and nutritious. In fact, no artificial sweetener can make such a claim, and all are controversial.

Neotame

In 2002, the FDA approved Neotame, a synthetic derivative of a combination of aspartic acid and phenylalanine, the same amino acids that are used to make aspartame. The difference between neotame and aspartame is that the bond between the amino acids in neotame is harder to break down making it more stable. Since our bodies can't metabolize neotame, only very small amounts are needed to sweeten foods and there is no danger to people suffering with PKU.

Neotame is promoted as a flavor enhancer, and the neotame web site states that it's safe for use by people of all ages, including pregnant or breastfeeding women, teens and children, and can be used in cooking. The FDA has set an acceptable daily intake (ADI) at 18 mg/kg of body weight/day.

Neotame entered the market more quietly than the other artificial sweeteners. While the web site for neotame claims there are over 100 scientific studies to support its safety, they are not readily available to the public. Opponents of neotame claim that the studies do not address the long-term health implications of using this sweetener. The chemical similarity of neotame to aspartame may mean that it can cause the same problems, but without scientifically sound studies done by independent labs, there's no way of knowing if, and for whom, this sweetener is safe.

Rebiana

Rebiana, rebaudioside A, or Reb-A, is a derivative of the stevia plant developed by Cargill, Inc., in partnership with The Coca-Cola Company and marketed by Cargill under the Truvia brand. A similar product, PureVia, was developed by PepsiCo in partnership with artificial sweetener industry veteran Merisant.

Based on several very short term studies funded exclusively by industry, Rebiana was added to the GRAS list in December 2008. The approval of Rebiana, however, was opposed by UCLA toxicologists and the CSPI, who reported that, while FDA's guidelines call for major new food additives to be tested for two years on both rats and mice, rebiana had only been tested on rats. The toxicologists and CSPI said that testing of rebiana in both rats and mice is particularly important because several tests found that rebiana-related substances caused mutations and damaged chromosomes or DNA.[166] In spite of the debates about rebiana's safety, the FDA approved the chemical and beverage companies started marketing rebiana-sweetened products.

Rebiana may be completely safe, but for now we will have to rely on assurances from its manufactures. No published studies have actually tested Truvia or PureVia themselves.

People who are allergic to ragweed may have an allergic reaction to stevia, of which Rebiana is a refined form.

Stevia

Stevia is obtained from a shrub that is grown in Brazil, Paraguay, southeast Asia, and elsewhere, and is about 100 times sweeter than sugar, The actual sweet chemicals are the closely related stevioside and rebaudioside A. Stevia and its derivatives are called "the holy grail" of high-potency sweeteners, because they are naturally derived alternatives to the controversial synthetic sweeteners saccharin, aspartame, acesulfame-K, sucralose and cyclamate.

In the 1990s, the U.S. FDA, Canada, and a European Community scientific panel declared that stevia was unacceptable for use in food and rejected stevia as a food ingredient.

High dosages of stevia fed to rats reduced sperm production and increased cell proliferation in their testicles, which could cause infertility or other problems. Pregnant hamsters that had been fed large amounts of a derivative of stevioside called steviol had fewer and smaller offspring. In the laboratory, steviol can be converted into a mutagenic compound, which may promote cancer by causing mutations in the cells' DNA.

Stevia is exempt under the FDA's GRAS policy due to its being a natural substance in wide use well before 1958. Unfortunately, there are no studies on the effects of this sweetener and the possible long-term consequences of children consuming it.

Tagatose

This sugar substitute is a synthetic additive chemically related to fructose. It does promote blood glucose or insulin levels but contains only about one third the calories of table sugar. It is not well-absorbed by the body and in large amounts can cause diarrhea, nausea, and flatulence.

Due to its bulk and sweetness, tagatose can be used in small amounts in baking and products subjected to high temperatures to increase the moistness and flavor, while maintaining sweetness. However, the processing and preparing of foods containing tagatose must accommodate certain temperature reactivity, as tagatose containing products "brown" and caramelize more readily than sucrose containing baked goods.

Artificial Sugars and Weight Gain

While most people who switch to artificial sugars do so to avoid the weight gain, there is significant evidence that there is a correlation between the ingestion of artificial sweeteners and weight gain.

The San Antonio Heart Study examined 3,682 adults over a seven- to eight-year period in the 1980s. When matched for initial body mass index (BMI), gender, ethnicity, and diet, drinkers of artificially sweetened beverages consistently had higher BMIs at the follow-up, with dose dependence on the amount of consumption. Average BMI gain was +1.01 kg/m2 for control and 1.78 kg/m2 for people in the third quartile for artificially sweetened beverage consumption. [167]

The American Cancer Society study conducted in the early 1980s included 78,694 women who shared the same similarities in age, ethnicity, socioeconomic status, and lack of preexisting conditions. A one-year follow-up showed 2.7 percent to 7.1 percent more regular artificial sweetener users gained weight compared to non-users matched by initial weight. The difference in the amount gained between the two groups was less than two pounds; nevertheless this was a significant number. [168]

In a recent study conducted by Purdue University researchers found that the intake of foods or fluids containing non-nutritive sweeteners was accompanied by increased food intake, body weight gain, accumulation of body fat, and weaker caloric compensation, compared to consumption of foods and fluids containing glucose.[169]

The Rudd Center for Food Policy and Obesity at Yale found that from 2006 to 2008, the number of advertisements children and teens saw for regular soda doubled. That's during a time when the American Beverage Association, the trade group for drink makers, said members had stopped advertising sugary drinks in children's programming.

The Rudd Center, which crusades for government regulation of food advertising and a tax on sugar-sweetened beverages, said the food industry spends more on marketing sweetened drinks to children than it does any other food category.

There are, of course, many factors involved in our national, and in the global, obesity epidemic. None of them, however, are even remotely as critical as sugar in our diets. Without targeting the huge and unnecessary amounts of sugar, both natural and artificial, that are currently being added to our food and drinks, we're not likely to make much progress. .

Eating in the Meantime

- The first step in reducing dietary sugar is reading those labels for sugar content. Be aware that one gram of (one teaspoon of white, granulated sugar) contains about 16 calories. Limit your child's sugar to six teaspoons a day. This doesn't include natural sugars found in fruit and milk.

- Using a variety of sweeteners will reduce your chances of ingesting significant amounts of any individual sweetener.

- A chart describing natural sweeteners is available in the Appendix. Many non-GM alternatives to high fructose corn syrup are available.

- When reading labels, look for the suffix –tol which denotes a sugar alcohol. Sugar alcohols are included in the amount of carbohydrates on the label but are not always listed separately as ingredients.

- The appendix also contains a list of Hidden Sugars, or sugars that may not be immediately identifiable within an ingredients list.

- Dog owners should take note that Xylitol can be toxic to dogs, even in small amounts. If your dog eats a product that contains xylitol, for example candy, it is crucial that you take the dog to a veterinarian immediately.

- Adequate data isn't available to establish aspartame's safety for children younger than 2, but few reasons exist, if any, to use a sugar substitute for children so young.

- Remember that sugar-free does not always mean zero sugar. Foods labeled "sugar free" must have less than 0.5 grams of sugar per serving. This means that you could actually ingest a fair amount of sugar if you eat more than a serving.

- Regardless of what they're called or how they're classified, sugar substitutes aren't magic bullets for weight loss. Take a closer look.

Chapter 11. Dangers in Our Daily Bread

For a lot of American consumers, even accustomed as we are to wild fluctuations in diet advice, the knowledge that there's something to worry about in plain old bread has come as a surprise. Bread, however, and the myriad products made of wheat have recently come under fire.

Many of us have known for a long time that white bread and refined grains in general aren't particularly nutritious. The aggressive processing of white flour leaves only a fraction of the nutrients of the original grain—the reason, as we discussed in Chapter 3, why commercial bread products are "fortified" or "enriched," often with synthetic micronutrients.

And, in Chapter 4, we learned about the variety of chemical additives that are a part of modern bread processing. But there's still another danger in the soft flour-bleaching process that creates soft white bread. Fewer of us know that the use of chlorine gas for bleaching of flours, a standard in the industry, produces a dangerous byproduct. That by-product is alloxan, a poison that is used to produce diabetes in healthy laboratory animals. Alloxan causes diabetes because it spins up enormous amounts of free radicals in pancreatic beta cells, thus destroying them.

White bread, however, is not the favorite it once was. Where only 15 years ago 80 percent of bread sold in the U.S. was white bread, today it's a much different story. We're buying more whole grain bread and less white, and in 2010, for the first time, sales of whole wheat bread surpassed that of white bread.[170]

This antipathy to bread is partly attributable to a growing

225

awareness of celiac disease, an autoimmune condition that affects approximately one in every 133 people. Celiac disease occurs when the small intestine is unable to properly digest gluten, a protein that appears in wheat as well as other grains such as barley, rye and spelt.

The increased occurrence of Celiac disease, has caused many to avoid bread, even if they don't have the disease. But the current anti-wheat trend isn't simply a response to celiac disease. Connections to other auto-immune diseases and implications for the obesity epidemic have cast modern wheat at least in a rather bad light.

What's Happened to Wheat?

For most of the ten thousand years that our ancestors cultivated wheat, this diet staple changed very little. Even after the grinding of wheat became mechanized in the early part of the twentieth century, the basic composition of flour was not appreciably different from the flour from which our ancestors made bread centuries before.

Indeed, the genetic distance that wheat has drifted since 1960 now exceeds the difference between chimpanzees and humans.

In the last half of the twentieth century, however, wheat began to undergo a radical transformation. Advancement in genetics allowed agricultural scientists to crossbreed and hybridize the wheat plant to increase yield and make it resistant to environmental conditions, pathogens and fungi. Compared to the slow, incremental breeding influences that occur in nature, the pace of these laboratory-designed changes have been incredibly rapid. The resulting "wheat" plant is something very far from what our ancestors, even our grandparents harvested. Indeed, the genetic distance that wheat has drifted since 1960 now exceeds the difference between chimpanzees and humans.

Wheat and Disease

Dr. William Davis has investigated the drastic transformation in wheat and believes that it has had serious effects on human health. His book, *Wheat Belly: Lose the Wheat, Lose the Weight, and Find Your Path Back to Health* published in 2011, created a sensation in indicting wheat particularly, and whole grains generally, as the food that was making us fat. Davis doesn't equivocate in tying wheat to the obesity epidemic. "I'd go as far," says Davis," as saying that overly enthusiastic wheat consumption is the *main* cause of the obesity and diabetes crisis in the United States." [171]

Whether or not you believe that heavy wheat consumption is the main cause or merely an important one of man, there's no question about the acceleration in wheat consumption corresponding to the acceleration in obesity.

Gluten-Related Disorders

The potential spectrum of so-called gluten-related disorders has expanded beyond the well-recognized and well-validated disorders of celiac disease.

Celiac Disease

Celiac disease is an autoimmune disorder in which gluten (a protein in wheat, barley, and rye, and sometimes in oats) causes the body's immune system to attack and damage the small intestine. It occurs in genetically predisposed people and can develop at any age but it is far more common in people with type 1 diabetes than in the general population. As many as 10 percent of children with type 1 diabetes, compared with only one in 100 children in the general population, test positive for the antibodies that indicate celiac disease. Moreover, a growing body of research suggests type 1 diabetes is also triggered by exposure to gluten, the protein linked to celiac disease, adding weight to the theory that the two disorders share common genetic causes.[172]

According to the Celiac Disease Foundation, celiac diseases estimated to affect 1 in 100 people worldwide. Two and one-half million Americans are undiagnosed and are at risk for long-term health complications.

Left untreated, celiac disease can lead to additional serious health problems. These include the development of other autoimmune disorders like Type I diabetes and multiple sclerosis (MS), dermatitis herpetiformis, anemia, osteoporosis, infertility and miscarriage, neurological conditions like epilepsy and migraines, short stature, and intestinal cancers.

Dermatitis Herpetiformis

Dermatitis Herpetiformis, also known as DH or Duhring's disease, is a skin manifestation of celiac disease. Itchy bumps or blisters appear on both sides of the body, most often on the forearms near the elbows, as well as on knees and buttocks.

The Celiac Disease Foundation estimates that DH affects 15 to 25 percent of people with celiac disease who typically have no digestive symptoms. DH can affect people of all ages, but most often appears for the first time in those between the ages of 30 and 40.

A skin biopsy is necessary to confirm a diagnosis of DH.

Gluten Sensitivity

It is now becoming clear that, besides Celiac Disease and wheat allergies, there are cases of gluten reactions in which neither allergic nor autoimmune mechanisms can be identified. These are generally defined as non-celiac Gluten Sensitivity. Some individuals who experience distress when eating gluten-containing products and show improvement when following a gluten-free diet may actually have Gluten Sensitivity instead. Gluten Sensitivity is a condition distinct from Celiac Disease and is not accompanied by the concurrence of anti-tTG autoantibodies or other autoimmune comorbidities. However, the two conditions cannot be distinguished clinically, since the symptoms experienced by Gluten Sensitive patients are often seen in

Celiac Disease.

While the small intestine of people with gluten sensitivity is usually normal, Gluten Sensitive individuals may have symptoms as severe as those of celiac disease. These symptoms include gastrointestinal distress, fatigue and headaches.

Wheat allergy

Wheat allergy is a separate disorder from gluten sensitivity. It can cause hives, skin rash, swelling of the lips and tongue, sneezing, watery eyes, difficulty breathing, and digestive symptoms.

Gluten-Free Labeling

A food product regulated by the FDA may be labeled gluten-free if it meets one of two conditions.

1). If it does NOT contain wheat, rye, barley or their crossbred hybrids like triticale (a gluten-containing grain),

OR

2) If it contains a gluten-containing grain or an ingredient derived from a gluten-containing grain that has been processed to less than 20 parts per million (ppm) of gluten.

These labeling rules, however, do not apply to foods regulated by the USDA. That means that meat, poultry and unshelled nuts are not covered. Nor are distilled spirits and wines that contain 7% or more alcohol by volume, or malted beverages made with malted barley or hops.

The Downsides of Gluten Free

For the many thousands of consumers who have lost weight and achieved near miraculous improvements in personal health, the issue of gluten vs. no gluten is well resolved. Yet even gluten-free evangelists will tell you that a gluten-free lifestyle is not always easy.

For one thing, going gluten-free can get expensive. Some commercially prepared gluten-free products can be two to three times more expensive than their gluten-containing counterparts. While there has been a definite explosion in gluten-free products entering the commercial market, you may still have a problem in finding safe-baking flours, mixes, dressings, and other gluten-free staples. It's a problem, however, that is rapidly correcting itself. Estimates for the US gluten-free retail market project a 38% to 48% growth rate by 2016.

An additional concern arises from the fact that many gluten-free foods are nutritionally inferior to their traditional counterparts. Commercially prepared gluten-free baked goods are often made with refined flours and starches (rice, potato, etc.) that are low in fiber and protein, and do not contain iron, folic acid and other B vitamins that are routinely added to wheat flour. Because most gluten-free grain products are not enriched, people with celiac can have a hard time getting enough of these key nutrients. Several studies have shown that people following a gluten-free diet, especially when relying on commercially prepared gluten-free foods, have diets low in iron, fiber, B vitamins, calcium and vitamin D.

Fortunately some manufacturers are beginning to use higher-fiber and more nutritious grains such as quinoa, amaranth, teff and sorghum. Manufacturers are also beginning to enrich gluten-free baked products with essential nutrients.

A last, but important worry for those watching their weight surrounds the starches that substitute for wheat flour in many gluten-free foods. Corn starch, rice starch, potato starch and tapioca starch are among the very few foods which increase blood sugar even more than wheat does.

Hidden Gluten

Gluten also shows up in many whole grain foods related to wheat, including bulgur, farro, kamut, spelt, and triticale (a hybrid of wheat and rye). Some celiac disease experts warn patients to steer clear of oats, as well.

A chart listing foods that signal the presence of gluten can be found in the Appendix. Other lists, and tips for discovering hidden gluten can be found on the website of The Celiac Disease Foundation (http://celiac.org).

Eating in the Meantime

- Apply the same scrutiny to products that claim to be gluten free that you would to any packaged food. Sometimes gluten-free versions have more added ingredients, especially sugar, than the regular ones.

- Recent studies conducted in Italy confirmed that tef, millet, amaranth, and quinoa were gluten free and found safe for the diets of patients with Celiac disease.

- There is no scientific evidence to suggest that products such as glutenase containing DPP-IV help those with celiac disease digest gluten. Save your money.

- The timing of our initial exposure to gluten as children is important, with infants fed gluten too early (2-4 months) show a far greater likelihood of developing celiac disease.

Chapter 12. The Fight For Real Food

For some of us, real food means only local, and seasonal. For others, only 100% USDA organic or Fair Trade deserves the name. We have some personal quibbles over exactly how fair, ecologically sound, humane, and community-based real food actually is. We're in agreement on what it's not.

It's not multi-sourced or highly processed. It's not chockfull of antibiotics or endocrine-disrupting hormones. It doesn't come from a CAFO or corporate industrial farm where animals are abused and human workers exploited. It doesn't have 3,000 miles of petroleum on it, and there isn't a patent on its seeds. It doesn't nourish us at the cost of irreparable damage to our planet and its natural resources. It doesn't deliberately conceal from us what it contains or how it's produced.

In short, real food is safe, healthy, and grown in ways that don't harm people or the planet. Unfortunately, that distinguishes it from the food that most of us eat most of the time. Perhaps our grandparents took real food for granted. Today's consumers can't. We need to fight for it. And we need to fight on many fronts.

The Fight for Organic Food

This book has addressed the many reasons why the fight for organic food is a fight for life in terms of both human wellbeing and the future of the planet. By now you know that organic is healthier for you and your children, and most of us think it's tastier too. You know that it keeps pesticides and chemicals off our plates and out of our bodies and also protects farm families, farm workers and surrounding communities from exposure to pesticide toxins. That it removes additional antibiotics from the food supply chain and doesn't contribute to the spread of GMOs. That organic production practices mitigate the effect of climate change through reduced reliance on fossil fuels and helps to safeguard our soil health and water supply.

Lots of us are now convinced of the immense benefits of organic food. Organic products have grown on average more than 20% per year over the last 7-10 years, making it the fastest growing segment of agriculture. That's the good news. But that growth doesn't necessarily mean that we can take the future of organic for granted. The food industry giants want in on that growth, too. In 1995 there were 81 independent organic processing companies in the United States. A decade later, Big Food had gobbled up all but 15 of them. These titans of processed food, junk food, and sugary beverages are the same companies who spend millions to defeat GMO labeling initiatives. The rapid consolidation of the organic industry means that small and medium size producers need our support more than ever.

As we learned in Chapter 3, the meaning of organic can also be undermined by manufacturers of conventional food who intentionally use marketing techniques to exploit consumer uncertainty about the term. This includes labeling conventional products as "organic" or trade-marking the word "organic" or "organics" as part of a brand name. The greatest threat to the organic label, however, may be coming from within.

There is significant pressure on the National Organic Program to relax organic standards and increasing concern that the USDA, overly friendly to corporate agribusiness, is abusing its authority by creating loopholes in enforcement of those standards. These abuses include reversing the "Sunset" provision which required the review of synthetic materials, allowing companies to petition for nanoparticles to be allowed in organic food, allowing giant, multimillion-dollar installations to grow plants indoors, under artificial lighting, and labeling the products *organic* without even identifying their origin as hydroponic, and more.[173] Such exemptions could quickly erode consumer confidence in organic foods and potentially destroy the industry.

The bottom line is that we must put our money and our principles where our values lie. We can do that by buying Certified Organic, not so-called natural products. Whenever possible, we can buy from the local or independent organic processor who is not likely to survive without our support. And we can tell our retail grocers that these are the products we want. Finally, as concerned consumers we must tell the USDA to use a public and transparent process for all major changes to organic standards. We need to tell our elected representatives how you feel and let them know you're paying attention. The integrity of the organic label is worth fighting for.

> The integrity of the organic label is worth fighting for.

The Fight for Local Food
and Community Agriculture

The fight for local food and community agriculture is a critical front in the Great American Food fight. It's one that goes well beyond securing fresher, healthier, and safer foods for your immediate family. It also means supporting animal welfare, protecting the planet, and working for economic justice for farmers. Local food systems help improve food security by making fresh food available to populations with limited access to healthful food. They support local economies and protect local farms and farmland. By employing sustainable practices, such as minimal pesticide use and no-till agriculture and composting, by reducing transport to consumers, and by minimizing or eliminating packaging for their farm products, many small-scale, local farms are helping to ameliorate the environmental damage done by industrial farming.

Fortunately the interest in local food production has been gathering steam recently. Even within bustling cities it's now possible to meet local farmers at farmers markets and obtain naturally raised meat and vegetables. And city farming itself has become part of the new food movement and a new green revolution that holds the promise of bringing real reform to our broken food system.

Urban farming comes in a variety of models. Some advocate the development of carefully controlled multi-story high-volume vertical farms that utilize the latest in aquaponic and hydroponic technologies. Other models of urban farming are lower-tech, using greenhouses and indoor and outdoor container gardening. Garden Labs, in New York and Philadelphia, uses these methods, while Common Good City Farm, in Washington, D.C., plants directly on its own acreage. Both programs also manage urban farming and education projects.

The success of programs like these, as well as the growth of farmer's markets and the explosion in windowsill and rooftop gardens all over the nation testify to what more and more of us have discovered. Just because we live in cities doesn't mean that our food can't be local.

As the farm-to-table movement evolves we're learning new ways to bring the farm much closer to the table. New online portals are helping to build a better food chain by connecting farmers and producers with food buyers, making the farm-to-table process seamless. By removing the middle man, portals like FarmersWeb.com enable farmers to cut down on costs, resulting in more local sourcing activity overall. Farm to Restaurant, Farm to Hospital, and Farm to School programs also now hold hope for shortening the food chain and getting fresher, healthier, safer food on our plates. Indeed, one particular movement, The Real Food Challenge, has made astonishing progress in a very short time. A grassroots activist group, Real Food Challenge developed a document called the Real Food Campus Commitment, which is presented to university presidents who are urged to sign on and promise that their schools will purchase at least 20 percent "real" (or sustainable) food by the year 2020. To date at least 134 colleges and universities have joined the program.

There's a lot that individuals and families can do in the fight for local food. We can buy from local farmers markets and from vegan, organic, and farm-to-table restaurants. We can join a food cooperative or subscription-based Community Supported Agriculture (CSA). We can volunteer to plant a community or school garden. We can work to urge local city governments to turn vacant land into urban gardens and support policies that encourage urban agriculture. And no matter where we live we can grow something to eat.

For local food, community agriculture and small, sustainable farming to have a real chance, however, we'll need reform in the halls of Congress. Americans must pressure our government to shift its support from corn and soy production, which supplies the production of processed foods and the factory farms that have wreaked so much havoc over the years, to smaller, ecological farms producing a diverse range of fruits and vegetables that supply their local and regional food systems and increase food security. The Great American Food Fight website provides information on contacting your elected representative, links to food issues that are coming before Congress, and to important organizations that are already fighting on our behalf.

When we combine our trip to the farmer's market or our CSA pickup with an email to our elected representative, we're delivering a real one-two punch. The fight for a rich, local food system is one in which every one of us can participate.

The Fight for Real School Food

Given what we know about soaring obesity rates in our children it seems self-evident that our schools must be a battleground in the fight for real food. First Lady Michelle Obama thought so, making childhood nutrition her signature issue. In 2010, the first lady championed the Healthy, Hunger-Free Kids Act, the largest investment in the National School Lunch Program in more than 30 years. The legislation aligned school meal requirements with USDA Dietary Guidelines and incorporated standards set by the Institute of Medicine.

Among other changes, the Act attempted to increase the amount and variety of fruits and vegetables served at meals by requiring kids to take at least one serving of either at meal time. It banned trans fats and set limits on saturated fats, required that water be free and accessible at meals, set calorie minimums and maximums based on age/grade groups, and set staged limits on sodium reduction.

These changes were championed by nutrition experts, by the American Heart Association, even a group of retired generals who think poor nutrition in schools has become a national security issue. Some of the new standards began phase-in in 2012, while others, like the lower sodium standards, had a 2017 deadline.

It didn't take long, though, for school lunches to become a political football and for Congress to begin undermining the standards. Opponents of the new standards claimed that students were rejecting and throwing away the healthier foods. A study published in the *American Journal of Preventive Medicine* found that food waste in studied schools was no greater after the reforms than before, and that vegetable consumption had increased by 16.2 percent,[174] but it came too late. Whole grain and sodium standards fell victim to the 2014 year-end spending bill.

There are lots of arguments against school food reform, the most hollow and hypocritical being that students should have the "freedom" to choose the food they want. Responsible parents, however, would no more allow their children to choose dinners of candy, ice cream and potato chips than they would allow them the freedom to play in a busy street. The freedom argument would be much more compelling if there actually *were* more real choices in school food. Free choice would be a cafeteria that offers nutritious selections well as fatty fried foods, and vending machines that offer fresh fruit in addition to Cheetos.

As Chapter One of this book outlines, the "freedom of choice" argument is meaningless if real choice doesn't exist, if we don't have the facts we need to make good choices, or if we're being unduly pressured in those choices. In the environment of many schools, where junk food marketing is emblazoned on books bags, vending machines, stadiums, and school buses and has invaded the classroom in the form of commercials for educational TV programming, there's a lot of pressure to make poor choices. Junk food marketing shouldn't be allowed to mask as education. Pupils aren't "targets," and the school day is not a market niche. As least in public school environments we should be able to offer our kids some protection from the onslaught of junk food and fast food huckstering.

Finally, the fight for real school food must address the desperate need for nutrition education and food literacy in the classroom. While the logos, licensed characters and products of fast food franchises are immediately recognizable to most kids, too many of them are completely disconnected from the nature and source of real food. Here in the U.S., school food activists like "lunch lady" Ann Cooper and celebrity chef Jamie Oliver have shocked us by revealing how many of our kids can't identify basic whole foods. It's a problem that exists all over the industrialized world. A U.K survey of 2,000 16- to 23-year-olds found that over half didn't know that butter comes from dairy cows, only two-thirds knew that eggs come from hens and over a third had no clue that bacon comes from pigs.

Fortunately, there are remedies for this disconnect which also bring real food to the classroom. The National Farm to School Network is one of our favorites. Students gain access to healthy, local foods as well as educational opportunities in the form of school gardens, cooking lessons and farm field trips. The program now involves 40,000 schools in all 50 states. Many non-profits are also working hard to promote better eating, nutrition education and environmental awareness in our schools. Ann Cooper's Chef Ann Foundation, Two Angry Moms, The Healthy Schools Campaign, The Edible Schoolyard, the Physicians for Responsible Medicine's Healthy School Lunch Campaign, and Wellness in the Schools are only a few. Links to these organizations and more can be found on the Great American Food Fight website.

We really <u>can</u> make progress in reversing the obesity epidemic and reducing national health costs. But we'll never do it by ignoring the place that 32 million children learn, and eat half their calories, every day. It's going to take a collective effort. But the fight for real school food is one we absolutely must win.

The Fight for Food Transparency

The fight for mandatory labeling of genetically modified foods is, of course, front and center in the fundamental struggle to know what we're buying and eating. You've heard a lot about the GMO labeling battle in this book and the organizations like **Just Label it** who are leading the fight. They have no intention of slowing down until this important battle is won. But the chokeholds that Big AG and Big Food have managed to clamp on the American diet mean that there are a lot of other areas where Americans are eating in the dark.

Some of these dark spots are other labeling issues, and pretty basic ones at that. The science is clear about the link between added sugars and the nation's obesity crisis. Consumers want to know how much sugar naturally occurs in a product and how much more has been added. And the FDA, over a year ago, proposed that manufacturers be required to list "added sugars" on labels. But big manufacturers, like General Mills, Cargill, Hormel and Schwan, as well as trade groups like the Grocery Manufacturers Association and the National Manufacturers Association want to see that it doesn't happen. The Dairy Institute of California would prefer that consumers not know how many teaspoons of sugar are added to flavored milk. The cranberry industry doesn't think consumers need to know how much added sweetening those tart cranberries need. The list goes on and on. And the influence, and enormous lobbying budgets, of these companies and trade groups could extend the FDA's plodding rule-making process by years unless the American consumer speaks out.

But labeling issues aren't the only place where transparency is a concern. Food transparency also means having the right to know how your food is made and handled. And we don't mean access to trade secret herbs and spices.

In the last few years, at the behest of the meat, dairy and egg industry, several state legislatures have sought to criminalize the exposure of animal mistreatment, unsafe working conditions and environmental problems at industrial agricultural operations. Named "Ag Gag" bills by *New York Times* food columnist Mark Bittman, these laws block whistleblowing, making it illegal to take video or photos on factory farms or to seek employment for the purpose of exposing animal abuse or food safety problems. In 2011 Ag Gag bills failed in Florida, Iowa, Minnesota and New York, but bills have been introduced in other states.

The fight for food transparency does, indeed, mean keeping watch over how honestly our food is labeled, but it also involves fighting to keep the lights on in American food production. All of us can help by supporting those organizations like the Humane Society and the Society for the Prevention of Cruelty to Animals (SPCA) in their efforts to fight Ag Gag laws. We can search out companies and brands that follow very strict animal welfare guidelines and buy from those retailers who are making transparency part of their brand.

One day soon, as more of us question the origins of our food and demand transparency not just for ingredients but for restaurant sourcing, labor and animal welfare practices, "it's none of your business" will become a completely unacceptable answer.

Eating in the Meantime

In the introduction to her wonderful book, *The Surprising Power of Family Meals*, author Miriam Weinstein asks this thought-provoking question:

> What if I told you there was a magic bullet—something that would improve your daily life, your children's chances of success in the world, your family's health, our values as a society? Something that is inexpensive, simple to produce, and within the reach of pretty much everyone?[175]

The "magic bullet," that Weinstein proposes is the simple routine of sitting down together as a family to eat—a disappearing custom, it would seem, in many American households. It's the singular suggestion for this book's final "Eating in the Meantime" section, but it may well be the most helpful one we've offered. We agree, unequivocally, with Weinstein that this simple practice may be as close as anything we have not just to a magic bullet for our own families, but for our entire society.

For many of us the testament to the power of family meals will be mostly anecdotal. It will come from cherished memories of holiday traditions, favorite recipes, and the communal sharing of experiences that occurs when we gather around the family table. Those of us who were lucky enough to grow up having regular, sit-down family meals take it as an article of faith that eating together made us "better" in many important ways. Now science is validating what we knew all along.

In 1993, the National Center on Addiction and Drug Abuse at Columbia University, known as CASA, undertook a study to determine if they could discover what factors differentiated those teens who took up destructive behaviors like the use of drugs, alcohol, and tobacco, from those who didn't. They talked to about 1,200 teens and their parents and included many variables in their interviews while factoring out race, class, and ethnicity. The results of the study came as a surprise to the researchers. The greatest predictor of kids' behavior—a more important predictor than church attendance or even school grades—was eating dinner with the family.

For every year since then, CASA has repeated its surveys and has continued to issue an annual report on "The Importance of Family Dinners." [176] The Center's surveys have consistently found that the more often children have dinners with their parents, the less likely they are to smoke, drink, or use drugs. Relationships between parents and children are better in families who eat together frequently. School grades are even better!

While eating together as a family can inoculate our children against these dangers, family meal times are also potent tools for addressing the health concerns that are at the heart of this book. Other research conducted on the subject of family meals has found that children and adolescents who share meals with their families at least three times per week are also less likely to be overweight, to eat unhealthy foods, or to be at risk for eating disorders. In addition, the kids were 24% more likely to eat healthy foods like fruits and vegetables, to eat breakfast and also more likely to take a multivitamin. The opportunities that eating together as a family afford for talking about food, transferring nutrition education to children, learning about food preparation, and even cooking, are additional advantages.

Simply put: frequent family dinners may be our single most important weapon in the Great American Food Fight.

Conclusion

The goal of "choosing" to eat healthily has never been more difficult or complex. As this book has attempted to show, far too many food choices have been taken out of our hands, those decisions made for us by an industrialized food system that is focused on profit, not human health. And the prospect of changing that system—so huge, so monopolistic, and so lucrative—seems daunting if not downright hopeless.

There's cause for concern, but not for despair. There is more serious interest in how food is produced today than there has ever been. Many flanks of the food movement are generating passionate enthusiasm and already hard at work restoring human values to a market that for far too long has only served corporate profit.

Many of us believe that we can grow a new food system. From the grassroots up. One that doesn't sacrifice human dignity and health, animal welfare, social justice and environmental sustainability. As we learn more ourselves and educate each other. As neighbor joins neighbor to write letters, sign petitions, attend meetings, and make our voices heard at the community, state, regional, and national levels. As we join with other concerned individuals to demand real food at our children's school cafeteria or college food service. As our own organizations combine with others to build more and bigger coalitions supporting farmland preservation, or fair trade, or the humane treatment of animals. As our numbers get bigger and our voices louder so that policy makers and industry leaders have to hear us and act on our behalf.

By combining our individual and collection actions we can begin to take back the right to our own choices and to restore democracy to our food system. We can make the food industry more honest and transparent. We can restore scientific integrity to food research and public health policy, and give our kids a fighting chance at good health and a long life.

We'll need to get smarter, get together, and get busy. We'll have to fight on many fronts. Most of us will have to pick a battle. But Americans are fighters and each of us can contribute. The future of food is the future of all of us. If you eat, this is your fight, too.

Appendix

BPA Free Products

Category	Product	Manufacturer
Infants and Toddlers	Baby bottles and nipples	• Born Free • Dr. Brown's • Green to Grow • Phillips Avent • Think Baby • Wee Go • Diapers Etc.
	Food and bottle warmer	• Phillips Avent
	Baby food maker	• Beaba Babycook
	Pacifiers and teethers	• Dano 2 • Diapers Etc • GumDrops • Natursutten • Razbaby • Soothie.
	Eating utensils	• Nuk • Green Eats • Learning Curve • Diapers Etc.
	Sippy cups	• Foogo • USA Kids • Bornfree • iPlay Babywear • Diapers Etc • Thinkbaby
	Bath toys	• Sassy • Greentoys • Boon
Canned Foods	All canned foods	• Eden Organic
	Meat products, fruits and vegetables	• Trader Joe's
	Tomatoes	• Muir Glen • Hunts
	Tomato paste, strained tomatoes	• Bionature
	All canned foods	• Native Forest/Native Factor

	Organic free range chicken broth; tomato soup	• Pacific Natural Foods
	Beans, fish, poultry, miscellaneous meat products, fruits and vegetables	• Trader Joe's
	Coconut milk	• Native Forest • Aroy-D • Trader Joe's
Seafood	Natural anchovy fillets; clam juice; natural clam juice; natural smoked baby clams in olive oil; natural skinless and boneless pink salmon; natural smoked Alaskan Coho salmon; natural albacore tuna (with and without salt); natural Tongol Tuna (with and without salt); yellowfin tuna in olive oil; yellowfin tuna in spring water' Albacore tuna	• Crown Prince • Ecofish • Starkist • VItal Choice Seafood • Wild Planet • Oregon's Choice
Cookware	Microwave cookware	• Pyrex • NordicWare • Corelle
Food and Water Containers	Food storage	• Rubbermaid • Snapware • Kinetic Go Green • Fit and Fresh • Farberware • Ziploc • Easy Lunchboxes • LockandLock
	Food wrap	• SC Johnson (Saran wrap)
	5 gallon water bottles	• Bluewave • Reliance Water-Pak • New Wave Enviro Products
	Water bottles	• Brita • Klean Kanteen • Nalgene • Camelbak • Campmor • Nalgene • Thermos • Rubbermaid
	Sports bottles	• No Sweat • Good Life Gear • Bluewave Bullet Hds Trading
	Water pitchers	• Brita • Rubbermaid
	Ice chests	• Rubbermaid • Igloo

Colorings and Dyes

Name	AKA	Approval	Uses	Health Risks	Notes
Blue 1	FD&C Blue No. 1, Brilliant Blue	Allowed	Found in pet food, beverages, candy, baked goods, icings, and syrups. Also used for personal care products.	Testing showed that male mice had a significant amount of kidney tumors in the mid-dose group. Causes occasional allergic reactions. Potential for neurotoxicity which affects fetuses and babies under the age of six months.	Banned in Norway, Finland, and France due to effect on allergic reactions in people with asthma. Overall production of this food dye in the U.S. exceeds 1 million pounds yearly.
Blue 2	IndigoCarmine	Allowed	Used to color beverages, candies, pet food and other food and drugs.	Inconclusive animal studies produced evidence of possible brain cancer in male rats. FDA conclusion is there is "reasonable certainty of no harm."	Experts maintain there is no convincing evidence of this dye's safety, and have called for discontinuing it in any products consumed by the general population.
Citrus Red 2	CI Solvent Red 80, CI 12156	Approval limited to coloring skins of oranges.	Found in the skin of some Florida oranges.	Toxic to rats and mice, even at a minimal level. According to the FDA, this dye is a bladder carcinogen.	The committee on food additives has stated that this color should not be used as a food additive.
Orange B	Azo Dye	Approval limited to use in hot dogs and sausage casings	Found in sausage casings and hot dogs.	High doses are harmful to the liver and bile duct. Animal studies showed that this dye affected the spleen, bile ducts, and urinary tracts. High doses of this dye killed rats.	The FDA proposed banning this dye in 1978, but because this dye has not been used for many years, the ban was never finalized, despite public outcries for doing so.
Red 3	Erythrosine	Allowed	Used to dye cherries, fruit cocktail, candy, and baked goods.	Has been shown to cause thyroid tumors in rats. Also used as a pesticide to kill flies' eggs (maggots) in manure piles (source: US EPA).	Replaced by Red 40, but still used in some foods such as cake icing, fruit roll-ups, and chewing gum. Banned in cosmetics and some drugs.
Green 3	Fast Green	Allowed	Personal care products, cosmetics except for eyes,	An industry-sponsored study linked this dye to bladder cancer in 1971, but the FDA, using other statistical tests, concluded that the dye	This dye is not widely used, however, recommendations have been made that this dye should

			beverages, sorbet, ingested drugs, lipsticks, and externally applied cosmetics.	was safe.	remain suspect until further tests have proven its safety.
Red 40	Allura Red AC, FD&C Red. No. 40	Allowed	The most widely used food color, this dye is used in sweets, drinks, children's medications, cereal, beverages, snacks, gelatin desserts , baked goods, and ice cream	Causes hypersensitivity in humans and triggers hyperactivity in children. Connected to cancer in mice. Developmental, reproductive, and general organ toxicity has also been noted in animal studies. Caution advised to those with aspirin sensitivities.	Banned in Denmark, Belgium, France, Germany, Switzerland, Sweden, Austria, and Norway. Recommendations have been made in the U.S. that Red 40 should not be used in foods.
Yellow 5	Tatrazine	Allowed	Found in gelatin, candy, pet food, and baked goods.	Causes allergy-like hypersensitivity reactions, primarily in aspirin-sensitive individuals. Can trigger hyperactivity in children.	Has not been adequately tested in mice, and serves no nutritional or safety purpose. Experts argue that it should not be allowed in the food supply.
Yellow 6	Sunset Yellow	Allowed	Used to color bakery goods, cereals, beverages, dessert powders, candies, gelatin, sausage, cosmetics, and drugs.	May cause occasional and severe hypersensitivity. May cause hyperactivity in some children. Animal tests show that this dye causes tumors of the adrenal gland and kidney. The FDA has reviewed data and concluded that this dye does not post a significant cancer risk to humans.	Banned in Norway and Sweden. Some evidence that dye may be contaminated with significant levels of recognized carcinogens. Recommendations have been made that because it provides no health benefit whatsoever, Yellow 6 should be removed from the food supply.

Cooking with Fats and Oils

Fat or Oil	Dressings and Dips	Heating	Stir Frying	Deep Frying	Baking	Note
Butter	Yes	Yes	Yes	Yes	Yes	
Canola	Yes		No	No	No	Usually GMO. Only use cold pressed or organic
Coconut	Yes	Yes	Yes	Yes	Yes	
Cottonseed						Usually GMO. Some allergy risk.
Corn			No		No	Usually GMO.
Flaxseed	Yes	Low temps only	No	No	Yes	
Grapeseed	Yes	Yes	Yes	Yes	Yes	
Margarine	No	No	No	No	No	Choose butter instead
Olive Oil	Yes	Low temps only	No	No		Preferably use extra virgin
Peanut			Yes			
Palm Kernel						
Lard	No	Yes	Yes	Yes	Yes	
Palm						
Safflower				No		Some allergy risk
Sesame						
Soybean						Usually GMO
Sunflower						

Smoke Points of Fats and Oils

Oil/Fat	Fahrenheit	Celsius
Canola Oil - Unrefined	225°F	107°C
Flaxseed Oil – Unrefined	225°F	107°C
Safflower Oil - Unrefined	225°F	107°C
Sunflower Oil - Unrefined	225°F	107°C
Corn Oil - Unrefined	320°F	160°C
Peanut Oil - Unrefined	320°F	160°C
Olive Oil – Unrefined	320°F	160°C
Soy Oil - Unrefined	320°F	160°C
Safflower Oil – Semi refined	320°F	160°C
Walnut Oil – unrefined	320°F	160°C
Butter	350°F	177°C
Canola Oil – Semi refined	350°F	177°C
Coconut Oil	350°F	177°C
Hemp Seed Oil	350°F	177°C
Sesame Oil - Unrefined	350°F	177°C
Soy Oil – Semi refined	350°F	177°C
Vegetable Shortening	350°F	177°C
Lard	360°F	
Walnut Oil, Semi-Refined	400°F	
Canola Oil - Refined	400°F	
Olive Oil - High Quality, Extra Virgin	405°F	206°C
Olive Oil - Virgin	420°F	215°C
Cottonseed Oil	420°F	215°C
Corn Oil - Refined	450°F	232°C
Peanut Oil - Refined	450°F	232°C
Safflower Oil - Refined	450°F	232°C
Sesame Oil – Semi refined	450°F	232°C
Soy Oil – Refined	450°F	232°C
Sunflower Oil - Refined	450°F	232°C
Canola Oil – Semi refined	465°F	240°C
Olive Oil - Extra Light	470°F	243°C
Canola Oil - Refined	470°F	243°C
Grapeseed Oil	485°F	
Avocado Oil - Refined	520°F	270°C

Safe Minimum Cooking Temperatures

Use this chart and a food thermometer to ensure that meat, poultry, seafood, and other cooked foods reach a safe minimum internal temperature.

Category	Food	Temperature (°F)	Rest Time
Ground Meat & Meat Mixtures	Beef, Pork, Veal, Lamb	160	None
	Turkey, Chicken	165	None
Fresh Beef, Veal, Lamb	Steaks, roasts, chops	145	3 minutes
Poultry	Chicken & Turkey, whole	165	None
	Poultry breasts, roasts	165	None
	Poultry thighs, legs, wings	165	None
	Duck & Goose	165	None
	Stuffing (cooked alone or in bird)	165	None
Pork and Ham	Fresh pork	145	3 minutes
	Fresh ham (raw)	145	3 minutes
	Precooked ham (to reheat)	140	None
Eggs & Egg Dishes	Eggs	Cook until yolk and white are firm	None
	Egg dishes	160	None
Leftovers & Casseroles	Leftovers	165	None
	Casseroles	165	None
Seafood	Fin Fish	145 or cook until flesh is opaque and separates easily with a fork.	None
	Shrimp, lobster, and crabs	Cook until flesh is pearly and opaque.	None
	Clams, oysters, and mussels	Cook until shells open during cooking.	None
	Scallops	Cook until flesh is milky white or opaque and firm.	None

Types of Food Ingredients

The following summary lists the types of common food ingredients, why they are used, and some examples of the names that can be found on product labels. Some additives are used for more than one purpose.

Types of Ingredients	What They Do	Examples of Uses	Names Found on Product Labels
Preservatives	Prevent food spoilage from bacteria, molds, fungi, or yeast (antimicrobials); slow or prevent changes in color, flavor, or texture and delay rancidity (antioxidants); maintain freshness	Fruit sauces and jellies, beverages, baked goods, cured meats, oils and margarines, cereals, dressings, snack foods, fruits and vegetables	Ascorbic acid, citric acid, sodium benzoate, calcium propionate, sodium erythorbate, sodium nitrite, calcium sorbate, potassium sorbate, BHA, BHT, EDTA, tocopherols (Vitamin E)
Sweeteners	Add sweetness with or without the extra calories	Beverages, baked goods, confections, table-top sugar, substitutes, many processed foods	Sucrose (sugar), glucose, fructose, sorbitol, mannitol, corn syrup, high fructose corn syrup, saccharin, aspartame, sucralose, acesulfame potassium (acesulfame-K), neotame
Color Additives	Offset color loss due to exposure to light, air, temperature extremes, moisture and storage conditions; correct natural variations in color; enhance colors that occur naturally; provide color to colorless and "fun" foods	Many processed foods, (candies, snack foods margarine, cheese, soft drinks, jams/jellies, gelatins, pudding and pie fillings)	(See Colors and Dyes Chart)
Flavors and Spices	Add specific flavors (natural and synthetic)	Pudding and pie fillings, gelatin dessert mixes, cake mixes, salad dressings, candies, soft drinks, ice cream, BBQ sauce	Natural flavoring, artificial flavor, and spices

Types of Ingredients	What They Do	Examples of Uses	Names Found on Product Labels
Flavor Enhancers	Enhance flavors already present in foods (without providing their own separate flavor)	Many processed foods	Monosodium glutamate (MSG), hydrolyzed soy protein, autolyzed yeast extract, disodium guanylate or inosinate
Fat Replacers (and components of formulations used to replace fats)	Provide expected texture and a creamy "mouth-feel" in reduced-fat foods	Baked goods, dressings, frozen desserts, confections, cake and dessert mixes, dairy products	Olestra, cellulose gel, carrageenan, polydextrose, modified food starch, microparticulated egg white protein, guar gum, xanthan gum, whey protein concentrate
Nutrients	Replace vitamins and minerals lost in processing (enrichment), add nutrients that may be lacking in the diet (fortification)	Flour, breads, cereals, rice, macaroni, margarine, salt, milk, fruit beverages, energy bars, instant breakfast drinks	Thiamine hydrochloride, riboflavin (Vitamin B_2), niacin, niacinamide, folate or folic acid, beta carotene, potassium iodide, iron or ferrous sulfate, alpha tocopherols, ascorbic acid, Vitamin D, amino acids (L-tryptophan, L-lysine, L-leucine, L-methionine)
Emulsifiers	Allow smooth mixing of ingredients, prevent separation, keep emulsified products stable, reduce stickiness, control crystallization, keep ingredients dispersed, and to help products dissolve more easily	Salad dressings, peanut butter, chocolate, margarine, frozen desserts	Soy lecithin, mono- and diglycerides, egg yolks, polysorbates, sorbitan monostearate
Stabilizers and Thickeners, Binders, Texturizers	Produce uniform texture, improve "mouth-feel"	Frozen desserts, dairy products, cakes, pudding and gelatin mixes, dressings, jams and jellies, sauces	Gelatin, pectin, guar gum, carrageenan, xanthan gum, whey
pH Control Agents and acidulants	Control acidity and alkalinity, prevent spoilage	Beverages, frozen desserts, chocolate, low acid canned foods, baking powder	Lactic acid, citric acid, ammonium hydroxide, sodium carbonate

Types of Ingredients	What They Do	Examples of Uses	Names Found on Product Labels
Leavening Agents	Promote rising of baked goods	Breads and other baked goods	Baking soda, monocalcium phosphate, calcium carbonate
Anti-caking agents	Keep powdered foods free-flowing, prevent moisture absorption	Salt, baking powder, confectioner's sugar	Calcium silicate, iron ammonium citrate, silicon dioxide
Humectants	Retain moisture	Shredded coconut, marshmallows, soft candies, confections	Glycerin, sorbitol
Yeast Nutrients	Promote growth of yeast	Breads and other baked goods	Calcium sulfate, ammonium phosphate
Dough Strengtheners and Conditioners	Produce more stable dough	Breads and other baked goods	Ammonium sulfate, azodicarbonamide, L-cysteine
Firming Agents	Maintain crispness and firmness	Processed fruits and vegetables	Calcium chloride, calcium lactate
Enzyme Preparations	Modify proteins, polysaccharides and fats	Cheese, dairy products, meat	Enzymes, lactase, papain, rennet, chymosin
Gases	Serve as propellant, aerate, or create carbonation	Oil cooking spray, whipped cream, carbonated beverages	Carbon dioxide, nitrous oxide

MSG Substitutes

Hydrolyzed Protein

Hydrolyzed Plant Protein

Hydrolyzed Vegetable Protein (HVP)

Plant Protein Extract

Sodium Caseinate

Calcium Caseinate

Yeast extract

Dried yeast

Torula yeast

Textured protein

Textured vegetable protein

Autolyzed yeast

Hydrolyzed oat flour

Corn oil

Food additives that frequently contain MSG

Malt extract

Malt flavoring

Bouillon

Broth

Stock

Flavoring

Natural flavors or flavoring

Natural beef flavoring

Natural chicken flavoring

Natural pork flavoring

Seasoning

Spices

Whey protein

Plastic Coding

1 PETE	**PET or PETE** (polyethylene terephthalate) containers are recyclable and safe for single use. But studies indicate that with repeated use, PET containers may release di(2-ethylhexyl) phthalate, an endocrine-disrupting compound and probable human carcinogen. PET bottled-water containers have also been found to leach the elemental metal antimony (an eye, skin and lung irritant at high doses), according to the January 2006 *Journal of Environmental Monitoring*. And in an animal study, rats that drank very low levels of antimony for most of their lives died sooner than rats that did not. Although the levels found fell within safe drinking-water standards, study author Bill Shotyk notes that concentrations in bottled water increase over time.
2 HDPE	**HDPE (high density polyethylene)** the thicker, milkier or opaque plastic found in milk and water jugs, juice bottles, detergent, shampoo, and motor oil containers, and toys. Safe to refill and reuse.
3 PVC	**Vinyl or PVC (polyvinyl chloride)**, which releases carcinogenic dioxins into the environment and can leach hormone-disrupting phthalate plasticizers. PVC contains chlorine, so its manufacture can release highly dangerous dioxins. If you must cook with PVC, don't let the plastic touch food. Also never burn PVC, because it releases toxins.
4 LDPE	**Vinyl or PVC (polyvinyl chloride)**, which releases carcinogenic dioxins into the environment and can leach hormone-disrupting phthalate plasticizers. PVC contains chlorine, so its manufacture can release highly dangerous dioxins. If you must cook with PVC, don't let the plastic touch food. Also never burn PVC, because it releases toxins.

5 PP	**PP (polypropylene)** Found in hard but flexible plastics, such as those used for ice cream and yogurt containers, drinking straws, syrup bottles, salad bar containers, and diapers. One of the safer plastics – but recycle, don't throw away.
6 PS	**PS (polystyrene)** Polystyrenes are familiar to us in coffee cups and to-go containers. Polystyrene can be made into rigid or foam products -- in the latter case it is popularly known as the trademark Styrofoam can leach styrene. The 12th Report on Carcinogens (June, 2011) issued by the Department of Health and Human Services lists styrene as a "possible human carcinogen."
7 OTHER	This category for miscellaneous plastics includes polycarbonate, a transparent plastic that contains hormone-disrupting bisphenol A, (BPA) which may stray into contents when stressed by heat or age. A wide variety of plastic resins that don't fit into the previous categories are lumped into number 7. A few are even made from plants (polyactide) and are compostable. Polycarbonate is number 7, and is the hard plastic that has parents worried these days, after studies have shown it can leach potential hormone disruptors.

Non-Dairy Sources of Calcium

Food	Serving Size	Calcium Amount (mg)
Dried Figs	4	506
Tofu (firm)	½ cup	434
Soy milk (fortified)	1 cup	400
Sardines w/bones	3 ounces	370
Sesame seeds	¼ cup	351
Rice milk (fortified)	1 cup	300
Fortified orange juice	1 cup	300
Fortified cereal	1 cup	300
Soy yogurt (vanilla)	1 6-ounce container	299
Canned salmon w/bones	4 ounces	285
Collard greens	1 cup	266
Spinach (boiled)	1 cup	245
Soy cheese (fortified)	1 ounce	200
Almond milk (fortified)	1 cup	200
Soybeans (cooked)	1 cup	180
Blackstrap molasses	1 Tbsp.	172
Tofu	4 ounces	154
Waffle (fortified)	1	150
Red kidney beans	½ cup	150
Shrimp	1 cup	147
Kelp (raw)	1 cup	136
Navy beans	1 cup	130
Tahini paste	1 tsp.	129
Turnip greens (cooked)	½ cup	124
Broccoli	2 cups	124
Black beans	1 cup	120
Apricots	4 small	117
Ocean Perch (Atlantic, cooked)	3 ounces	116
Oatmeal (plane and flavored, instant, fortified)	1 packet	110
Cowpeas (cooked)	½ cup	106
Swiss chard (boiled)	1 cup	102
Mustard greens	½ cup	100
White beans (canned)	½ cup	96
Kale (boiled)	1 cup	94
Brazil nuts	2 ounces (12 nuts)	90
Soybeans (mature, cooked)	½ cup	88

Okra (cooked from frozen)	½ cup	88
Blue crab (canned)	3 ounces	86
Beet greens (cooked fresh)	½ cup	82
Celery	2 cups	81
Oysters	3 ounces	80
Bok Choy	½ cup	80
Pak-Choi (Chinese cabbage)	½ cup	79
Clams (canned)	3 ounces	78
Garbanzo beans (canned)	1 cup	77
Almonds	1 ounce (23 nuts)	75
Sweet Potato (cooked)	1 cup	76
Dandelion greens (cooked fresh)	½ cup	74
Rainbow trout (farmed, cooked)	3 ounces	73
Papaya	1 medium	73
Soy milk (unfortified)	1 cup	61
Whole-wheat bread	2 slices	60
Carrot juice	1 cup	57
Oranges	1 medium	52
Flax seeds	2 Tbsp.	52
Flour or corn tortilla	1 6-inch	45
Green peas	1 cup	45
Almond butter	1 Tbsp.	43

Needed calcium intake according to age:
Ages 1-3 – 500 mg
Ages 4-8 – 800 mg
Ages 9-49 – 1000 mg
Ages 50 and above – 1200 mg

Non-Meat Sources of Protein

Dairy				
Name	**Serving Size**	**Protein Total Grams**	**Total Calories**	**Fat Total Grams**
American cheese	1 oz.	6	106	9
Blue cheese	1 oz.	6	100	8
Cheddar cheese	1 oz.	7	114	9
Cheddar/Colby , low-fat	1 oz.	7	49	2
Cottage cheese – fat-free	1 cup	31	160	1
Cottage cheese – 2% -	1 cup	30	203	4
Cottage cheese – 1%	1 cup	28	163	2
Feta cheese	1 oz.	4	75	6
Goat cheese	1 oz.	5	78	6
Mozzarella cheese – part skim	1 oz.	7	72	5
Parmesan cheese	1 oz.	12	129	9
Provolone cheese	1 oz.	7	100	8
Ricotta cheese – part skim	1 oz.	3	39	2
Swiss cheese	1 oz.	8	106	8
Goat's milk	1 cup	9	168	10
Milk – whole	1 cup	8	146	8
Milk – 2%	1 cup	8	121	7
Milk – 1%	1 cup	8	102	8
Milk – skim	1 cup	8	80	0
Yogurt – whole milk –	1 cup	9	150	8
Yogurt – plain – low-fat	1 cup	13	155	4
Yogurt – plain – fat-free	1 cup	14	137	0

Eggs				
Name	**Serving Size**	**Protein Total Grams**	**Total Calories**	**Fat Total Grams**
Egg (cooked or fried)	1	6	90	8
Egg (hard-boiled)	1	6	77	5
Egg white (cooked)	1	17	17	0
Egg substitute	¼ cup	5	30	0

Grains					
Name	**Serving Size**	**Protein Total Grams**	**Total Calories**	**Fat Total Grams**	**Fiber Total Grams**
Amaranth	1 cup cooked	9	251	4	9
Barley	1 cup cooked	4	198	1	14
Buckwheat	1 cup cooked	6	156	5	5
Brown rice	1 cup cooked	5	216	2	7
Bulgar	1 cup cooked	6	151	0	8
Oats	1 cup cooked	6	166	4	4
Quinoa	1 cup cooked	8	222	4	4
Spelt	1 cup cooked	11	246	2	4
Sprouted grain bread	1 slice	4	80	1	3
Whole wheat bread	1 slice	4	128	3	3
Whole wheat pasta	1 cup cooked	7	160	1	6

Legumes

Name	Serving Size	Protein Total Grams	Total Calories	Fat Total Grams	Fiber Total Grams
Black beans	1 cup cooked	15	227	1	15
Garbanzo beans (chickpeas)	1 cup cooked	15	269	4	12
Kidney beans	1 cup cooked	15	225	0	11
Lentils	1 cup cooked	18	230	1	16
Lima beans	1 cup cooked	15	216	1	13
Navy beans	1 cup cooked	16	258	1	12
Pinto beans	1 cup cooked	15	234	1	15
Split peas	1 cup. cooked	16	231	1	16
Soybeans	1 cup cooked	29	310	16	10

Nuts

Name	Serving Size	Protein Total Grams	Total Calories	Fat Total Grams	Fiber Total Grams
Dry roasted almonds	¼ cup	8	206	18	4
Hazelnuts	¼ cup	5	212	21	3
Pine nuts	¼ cup	5	229	23	1
Pistachios	¼ cup	6	171	14	3
Raw cashews	¼ cup	5	197	16	2
Raw peanuts	¼ cup	9	207	18	2
Walnuts	¼ cup	4	164	16	2

Seeds

Name	Serving Size	Protein Total Grams	Total Calories	Fat Total Grams	Fiber Total Grams
Flaxseed	¼ cup	8	224	18	12
Hemp seeds	¼ cup	11	162	10	1
Pumpkin seeds	¼ cup roasted	3	71	3	4
Sesame seeds	¼ cup roasted	6	182	15	6
Sunflower seeds	¼ cup	8	207	19	4

Soy

Name	Serving Size	Protein Total Grams	Total Calories	Fat Total Grams	Fiber Total Grams
Edamame	1 cup shelled	20	240	10	10
Soybeans	1 cup cooked	29	298	10	8
Soymilk (sweetened)	1 cup	7	100	0.5	3
Soymilk (unsweetened)	1 cup	7	80	0.5	2
Soy nuts	¼ cup roasted	11	200	1	3.5
Soy nut butter	2 Tbsp.	7	170	11	3
TVP	¼ cup dry	12	80	0	4
Tempeh	4 oz.	21	223	13	10
Tofu	4 oz.	9	86	5	1

Hidden Sugars

Agave Nectar
Barley Malt
Barley Malt Syrup
Beet Sugar
Blackstrap Molasses
Brown Rice Syrup
Brown Sugar
Cane Crystals
Cane Juice Crystals
Cane Sugar
Caramel
Castor Sugar
Carob Syrup
Coconut Sugar, or Coconut Palm Sugar
Confectioner's sugar
Corn Sugar
Corn Sweetener
Corn Syrup, or corn syrup solids
Crystalline Fructose
Date Sugar
Dehydrated Cane Juice
Demerara Sugar
Dextran
Dextrose
Diastatic Malt
Diatase
Ethyl Maltol
Evaporated Cane Juice
Fructose
Fructose glucose syrup
Fruit Juice
Fruit juice concentrate
Galactose
Glucose or glucose solids
Golden, sugar, golden syrup
Granulated sugar

Grape sugar
HFCS
High-fructose Corn Syrup
Honey Hydrogenated Starch
Hydrolysate (HSH)
Invert sugar
Lactose
Maltitol
Maltodextrin
Malt Syrup
Maltose
Maple Syrup
Molasses
Monk Fruit
Muscovado Sugar
Oligofructose
Palm Sugar
Panocha
Raw Sugar
Refiner's Syrup
Rice Syrup
Saccharose
Sorbitrol
Sorghum or sorghum syrup
Sucrulose
Sucrose
Syrup
Tagatose
Treacle
Trehalose
Turbinado Sugar
Xylitol
Xylose
Yacon Syrup
Yellow Sugar

Natural Sweeteners

According to the American Diabetes Services, these are some healthy alternatives to sugar and artificial sweeteners.

Raw Honey – Raw honey is packed with antioxidants, minerals, vitamins, amino acids, enzymes, carbohydrates and phytonutrients. Avoid the processed honey you see in the grocery store. It's stripped of these nutrients and it's no better than white table sugar. Some types of honey, such as red clover honey or orange blossom honey have a lower glycemic index.

Agave Nectar - Sweeter than honey, agave nectar is a combination of fructose and glucose sugars. This syrup is obtained by extracting and purifying the sap of the blue agave plant and is popular in both hot and cold drinks. In addition, agave nectar has a low glycemic index, so it does not have much effect on blood sugar levels.

Maple Syrup - This naturally-occurring sweetener is another excellent substitute for refined sugar. High in trace minerals like zinc and manganese, maple syrup can help balance cholesterol levels. It does, however, have a fairly high glycemic index so diabetics should be aware of this and use it moderately.

Brown Rice Syrup - While far less refined than table sugar, this sweetener is approximately 45% maltose, a type of sugar with a high glycemic index value. If you have diabetes, be sure to read the nutrition label and if this ingredient is listed, avoid it if possible.

Barley Malt Syrup – A natural sugar substitute; made by barley grains, which produces a type of sugar known as maltose. This sweetener is about half as sweet as refined sugar, has a molasses-like flavor and a distinctive rich, dark color. It's popular for use in cooking, baking and brewing beer. However, barley malt syrup is 65% maltose, which is high on the glycemic index, so diabetics should check the nutrition label when consuming products or baked goods with this sweetener.

Evaporated Cane Juice - This natural sugar does not undergo the same degree of processing that refined sugar does, so it retains more of the nutrients found in sugar cane. When consumed in moderation, evaporated cane juice is a natural source of sweetness that can be a part of a healthy diet. It can be used just like sugar to sweeten foods and beverages. Nutrition labels may list it by other names such as dried cane juice, crystallized cane juice or milled cane sugar.

Black Strap Molasses - When sugar cane is processed, its juice is extracted and boiled three times. The first boiling produces the crystallized sugar we know as table sugar. Black strap molasses is the concentrated byproduct of the third boiling and contains nutrients such as iron, calcium, copper, magnesium, manganese and potassium. This sweetener is a popular alternative to refined brown sugar in baked goods and baked beans.

Unsulphured molasses - Not only delivers a naturally sweet taste, but contains natural potassium, calcium and iron.

Organic Sugar – Organic sugar is derived from sugar cane that's grown without chemicals or pesticides. It's darker in color than table sugar because it isn't processed in the same way as white sugar, and it contains some molasses.

Sources of Gluten

Abyssinian Hard (Wheat triticum durum), Alcohol (Spirits - Specific Types), Atta (chapati flour)

Barley (flakes, flour, pearl, grass, seeds), Beer (most contain barley or wheat), Bleached Flour, Bran, Bread Flour, Brewer's Yeast, Brown Flour Breading, bread stuffing, Brewer's yeast, Bulgur (wheat, nuts)

Cereal Binding, Chilton. Club Wheat (Triticum aestivum subspecies compactum), Common Wheat (Triticum aestivum). Couscous. Criped Rice

Dinkle (Spelt), Disodium Wheatgermamido Peg-2 Sulfosuccinate, Durum wheat (Triticum durum)

Edible Starch, Einkorn (Triticum monococcum), Emmer (Triticum dicoccon)

Farina, Farro/faro (also known as spelt or dinkel), Fu (a dried gluten product made from wheat and used in some Asian dishes)

Graham flour, Granary Flour , Groats (barley, wheat)

Hard Wheat, Heeng,Hing, Hordeum Vulgare Extract, Hydroxypropyltrimonium, Hydrolyzed wheat protein

Kamut (type of wheat), Kecap Manis (Soy Sauce),Ketjap Manis (Soy Sauce),Kluski Pasta

Maida (Indian wheat flour), Malt, malt extract, malt syrup, malt flavoring, Malt vinegar, Malted Barley Flour, Malted milk, Matzo, matzo meal, Matzo Semolina, Meripro 711, Mir, Modified wheat starch

Oatmeal, oat bran, oat flour, whole oats (unless they are from pure, uncontaminated oats), Oriental Wheat (Triticum turanicum), Orzo Pasta

Pasta, Pearl Barley, Persian Wheat (Triticum carthlicum) ,Perungayam, Poulard Wheat (Triticum turgidum), Polish Wheat (Triticum polonicum) Rice Malt (if barley or Koji are used), Roux, Rusk,Rye, Rye bread and flour

Seitan (a meat-like food derived from wheat gluten used in many vegetarian dishes)
Semolina, Spelt (type of wheat also known as farro, faro, or dinkel), Sprouted Wheat or Barley, Stearyldimoniumhydroxypropyl Hydrolyzed Wheat Protein, Strong Flour,Suet in Packets

Tabbouleh ,Tabouli,Teriyaki Sauce,Timopheevi Wheat (Triticum timopheevii) Triticale , Triticum Vulgare (Wheat) Flour Lipids, Triticum Vulgare (Wheat) Germ Extract, Triticum Vulgare (Wheat) Germ Oil

Udon (wheat noodles),Unbleached Flour

Vavilovi Wheat (Triticum aestivum),Vital Wheat Gluten,

Wheat, Abyssinian Hard triticum durum, Wheat Amino Acids, Wheat Bran Extract, Flour, Germ, Oil, Protein. Wheat Grass (can contain seeds), Wheat Nuts, Wheat Protein, Wheat Triticum aestivum, Wheat Triticum Monococcum, Wheat (Triticum Vulgare) Bran Extract, Whole-Meal Flour,Wild Einkorn (Triticum boeotictim), Wild Emmer (Triticum dicoccoides)

References

1.   Prevention, C.f.D.C.a., *Vital Signs: Obesity Among Low-Income, Preschool-Aged Children — United States, 2008–2011*, in *Morbidity and Mortality Weekly Report*. 2015, Centers for Disease Control and Prevention.

2.   Ogden, C.L., et al., *Prevalence of childhood and adult obesity in the united states, 2011-2012.* JAMA, 2014. **311**(8): p. 806-814.

3.   Sturm, R. and A. Hattori, *Morbid obesity rates continue to rise rapidly in the United States.* Int J Obes, 2013. **37**(6): p. 889-891.

4.   Skinner, A.C. and J.A. Skelton, *Prevalence and trends in obesity and severe obesity among children in the United States, 1999-2012.* JAMA Pediatr, 2014. **168**(6): p. 561-6.

5.   Press, T.N.A., *U.S. Health in International Perspective: Shorter Lives, Poorer Health*, ed. H.W. Steven and A. Laudan. 2013: The National Academies Press.

6.   Farrell, G.C., *The liver and the waistline: Fifty years of growth.* J Gastroenterol Hepatol, 2009. **24 Suppl 3**: p. S105-18.

7.   Fund, U.S.P.E. *Apples to Twinkies: Comparing Federal Subsidies of Fresh Product and Junk Food.* 2011.

8.   Robinson, T.N., et al., *Effects of Fast Food Branding on Young Children's Taste Preferences.* Arch Pediatr Adolesc Med, 2007. **161**(8): p. 792-797.

9.   Roberto, C.A., et al., *Influence of licensed characters on children's taste and snack preferences.* Pediatrics, 2010. **126**(1): p. 88-93.

10.   Education, C.f.C.F. *Commercialism in Our Schools.* 2012 [cited 2012 July 16, 2012]; Available from: http://www.ibiblio.org/commercialfree/commercialism.html.

11.   Simon, M., *Appetite for Profit*, in *How the Food Industry Undermines Our Health and How to Fight Back.* 2006, Nation Books: New York.

12.   Makely, W., *Cost-savings start with accurate analysis of actual per-package costs: the complex factors that affect packaging costs resist reduction to a single formula. Experience, both human and economic, has to be part of the equation - Per-Package Cost Analysis.* Food & Drug Packaging, 2003(March).

13.   *Deloitte 2011 Consumer Food and ProductInsights Survey Part Two Slides_071911.pdf>.* 2011.

14.   *Air to spare.* Consumer Reports, 2010. **75**(1): p. 16-18.

15.   Irmak, C., B. Vallen, and S.R. Robinson, *The Impact of Product Name on Dieters' and Nondieters' Food Evaluations and Consumption.*

Journal of Consumer Research, 2011. **38**(2): p. 390-405.

16. Wansink, B., *How Do Front and Back Package Labels Influence Beliefs About Health Claims?* Journal of Consumer Affairs, 2003. **37**(2): p. 305-316.

17. Office, U.S.G.A., *<GAO Report on Health Claims.pdf>*. 2011: p. 60.

18. Nestle, M. and D.S. Ludwig, *Front-of-Package Food Labels.* JAMA: Journal of the American Medical Association, 2010. **303**(8): p. 771-772.

19. Nestle, M., *Food Politics: How the Food Industry Influences Nutrition and Health.* 2002, Los Angeles: University of California Press

20. Roberto, C.A., et al., *Choosing front-of-package food labelling nutritional criteria: how smart were 'Smart Choices'?* Public Health Nutr, 2012. **15**(2): p. 262-7.

21. Schuldt, J.P., D. Muller, and N. Schwarz, *The "Fair Trade" Effect: Health Halos From Social Ethics Claims.* Social Psychological and Personality Science, 2012.

22. Prevention, C.f.D.C.a. *CDC - NBP - Factsheet - BPA.* 2015 [cited 2015 2/18]; CDC Fact Sheet on Bisphenol A]. Available from: http://www.cdc.gov/biomonitoring/BisphenolA_FactSheet.html.

23. Rudel, R.A., et al., *Food packaging and bisphenol A and bis(2-ethyhexyl) phthalate exposure: findings from a dietary intervention.* Environ Health Perspect, 2011. **119**(7): p. 914-20.

24. Feskanich D, S.V.W.W.C.C.G.A., *VItamin a intake and hip fractures among postmenopausal women.* JAMA: The Journal of the American Medical Association, 2002. **287**(1): p. 47-54.

25. *Keep the Multi, Skip the Heavily Fortified Foods.* The Nutrition Source 2012 July 28, 2012 Available from: http://www.hsph.harvard.edu/nutritionsource/what-should-you-eat/folic-acid/#folic-acid.

26. Silverglade, B., and Ringel Heller, *Food Labeling Chaos Report*, C.f.S.i.t.P. Interest, Editor. 2010.

27. Brownell, K.D. and J.P. Koplan, *Front-of-package nutrition labeling-- an abuse of trust by the food industry?* N Engl J Med, 2011. **364**(25): p. 2373-5.

28. *AZODICARBONAMIDE.* Concise International Chemical Assessment Document 16 1999 November 9, 2012 [cited 2012 November 9, 2012]; Available from: http://www.inchem.org/documents/cicads/cicads/cicad16.htm.

29. McCann, D., et al., *Food additives and hyperactive behaviour in 3-year-old and 8/9-year-old children in the community: a randomised,*

double-blinded, placebo-controlled trial. Lancet, 2007. **370**(9598): p. 1560-7.

30. Tobacman, J.K., *Carrageenan Sunset Review*, in *National Organics Standard Board*. 2012: Washington, D.C.

31. Freeman, M., *Reconsidering the effects of monosodium glutamate: a literature review.* J Am Acad Nurse Pract, 2006. **18**(10): p. 482-6.

32. Hermanussen, M. and J.A. Tresguerres, *Does high glutamate intake cause obesity?* J Pediatr Endocrinol Metab, 2003. **16**(7): p. 965-8.

33. Insawang, T., et al., *Monosodium glutamate (MSG) intake is associated with the prevalence of metabolic syndrome in a rural Thai population.* Nutr Metab (Lond), 2012. **9**(1): p. 50.

34. Hermanussen, M., et al., *Obesity, voracity, and short stature: the impact of glutamate on the regulation of appetite.* Eur J Clin Nutr, 2006. **60**(1): p. 25-31.

35. Afifi, M.M. and A.M. Abbas, *Monosodium glutamate versus diet induced obesity in pregnant rats and their offspring.* Acta Physiol Hung, 2011. **98**(2): p. 177-88.

36. *MUltiple outbreaks of gastrointestinal illness among school children associated with consumption of flour tortillas—massachusetts, 2003-2004.* JAMA: The Journal of the American Medical Association, 2006. **295**(11): p. 1240-1246.

37. Ohno, Y., et al., *[Carcinogenicity of potassium bromate in F-344 rats].* Eisei Shikenjo Hokoku, 1982(100): p. 93-100.

38. Feingold, B.F., *Behavioral disturbances linked to the ingestion of food additives.* Del Med J, 1977. **49**(2): p. 89-94.

39. Feingold, B.E., *Feingold diet.* Aust Fam Physician, 1980. **9**(1): p. 60-1.

40. Stevenson, J., *Recent Research on Food Additives: Implications for CAMH.* Child and Adolescent Mental Health, 2010. **15**(3): p. 130-133.

41. Price, W.A., *Nutrition and physical degeneration.* 8th ed. 2008, La Mesa, CA: Price-Pottenger Nutrition Foundation. xxxvii, 527 p.

42. Enig, M.G., *Know your fats : the complete primer for understanding the nutrition of fats, oils and cholesterol.* 2000, Silver Spring, MD: Bethesda Press. xvi, 334 p.

43. Ravnskov, U., *The questionable role of saturated and polyunsaturated fatty acids in cardiovascular disease.* J Clin Epidemiol, 1998. **51**(6): p. 443-60.

44. Ravnskov, U. *My life and my work.* 2008 November 30, 2008 [cited 2012 12/10/2012]; Available from: http://www.ravnskov.nu/lifeandwork.htm.

45. Taubes, G., *What if It's All Been a Big Fat Lie?*, in *The New York Times*. 2002: New York. p. 1.

46. Parodi, P.W., *Has the association between saturated fatty acids, serum cholesterol and coronary heart disease been over emphasized?* International Dairy Journal, 2009. **19**(6-7): p. 345-361.

47. Volk, M.G., *An examination of the evidence supporting the association of dietary cholesterol and saturated fats with serum cholesterol and development of coronary heart disease.* Altern Med Rev, 2007. **12**(3): p. 228-45.

48. Castelli, W.P., *Concerning the possibility of a nut.* Arch Intern Med, 1992. **152**(7): p. 1371-2.

49. Eades, D.M.R. *Framingham Follies*. 2006 [cited 2013 January 8, 2013]; Available from: http://www.proteinpower.com/drmike/cardiovascular-disease/framingham-follies/.

50. Ascherio, A., et al., *Dietary fat and risk of coronary heart disease in men: cohort follow up study in the United States.* BMJ, 1996. **313**(7049): p. 84-90.

51. Howard, B.V., et al., *Low-fat dietary pattern and risk of cardiovascular disease: the Women's Health Initiative Randomized Controlled Dietary Modification Trial.* JAMA, 2006. **295**(6): p. 655-66.

52. Siri-Tarino, P.W., et al., *Meta-analysis of prospective cohort studies evaluating the association of saturated fat with cardiovascular disease.* Am J Clin Nutr, 2010. **91**(3): p. 535-46.

53. Donaldson, C., *The Rise and Fall of Trans Fat: Is the Battle Won?* Perspectives in Public Health, 2009. **129**(2): p. 57-58.

54. Calder, P.C., *Old study sheds new light on the fatty acids and cardiovascular health debate.* BMJ, 2013. **346**: p. f493.

55. Sauer, F.D., et al., *Additional vitamin E required in milk replacer diets that contain canola oil.* Nutrition Research, 1997. **17**(2): p. 259-269.

56. Coutinho, E.M., *Gossypol: a contraceptive for men.* Contraception, 2002. **65**(4): p. 259-263.

57. Yanagi, S. and M. Sakamoto, *Effect of Safflower Oil and Safflower Margarine on Hepatic Tumorigenesis by N N'-2 7 Fluorenylene Bis Acetamide.* Journal of Nara Medical Association, 1982. **33**(6): p. 443-594.

58. Michael Jacobson, P.D. *Statement on FDA Approval of Olestra.* 1996 January 24, 1996 [cited 2012 11/28/2012]; Press Release]. Available from: http://www.cspinet.org/new/olest1.html.

59. Daniel, C.R., et al., *Trends in meat consumption in the USA.* Public

Health Nutr, 2011. **14**(4): p. 575-83.

60.   Bottemiller, H. *Dispute over Drug in Feed, Limiting US Exports*. 2013 February 22, 2013 [cited 2013 March 12, 2013]; Available from: http://www.nbcnews.com/business/dispute-over-drug-feed-limiting-us-meat-exports-174014?streamSlug=businessmain.

61.   Authority, E.F.S., *<Safety Evaluation of Ractopamine.pdf>*. EFSA Journal, 2009. **1041**: p. 1-52.

62.   Bao, P.P., et al., *Fruit, vegetable, and animal food intake and breast cancer risk by hormone receptor status*. Nutr Cancer, 2012. **64**(6): p. 806-19.

63.   Swan, S.H., et al., *Semen quality of fertile US males in relation to their mothers' beef consumption during pregnancy*. Hum Reprod, 2007. **22**(6): p. 1497-502.

64.   Mouritsen, A., et al., *Hypothesis: exposure to endocrine-disrupting chemicals may interfere with timing of puberty*. Int J Androl, 2010. **33**(2): p. 346-59.

65.   Massart, F. and G. Saggese, *Oestrogenic mycotoxin exposures and precocious pubertal development*. Int J Androl, 2010. **33**(2): p. 369-76.

66.   Daley, C.A., et al., *A review of fatty acid profiles and antioxidant content in grass-fed and grain-fed beef*. Nutr J, 2010. **9**: p. 10.

67.   Sinha, R., et al., *Meat intake and mortality: a prospective study of over half a million people*. Arch Intern Med, 2009. **169**(6): p. 562-71.

68.   Pan, A., et al., *Red meat consumption and mortality: results from 2 prospective cohort studies*. Arch Intern Med, 2012. **172**(7): p. 555-63.

69.   Larsson, S.C. and A. Wolk, *Meat consumption and risk of colorectal cancer: a meta-analysis of prospective studies*. Int J Cancer, 2006. **119**(11): p. 2657-64.

70.   Faramawi, M.F., et al., *Consumption of different types of meat and the risk of renal cancer: meta-analysis of case-control studies*. Cancer Causes Control, 2007. **18**(2): p. 125-33.

71.   Larsson, S.C., N. Orsini, and A. Wolk, *Processed meat consumption and stomach cancer risk: a meta-analysis*. J Natl Cancer Inst, 2006. **98**(15): p. 1078-87.

72.   Wang, C. and H. Jiang, *Meat intake and risk of bladder cancer: a meta-analysis*. Med Oncol, 2011.

73.   Micha, R., S.K. Wallace, and D. Mozaffarian, *Red and processed meat consumption and risk of incident coronary heart disease, stroke, and diabetes mellitus: a systematic review and meta-*

analysis. Circulation, 2010. **121**(21): p. 2271-83.

74.   Peters, J.M., et al., *Processed meats and risk of childhood leukemia (California, USA).* Cancer Causes Control, 1994. **5**(2): p. 195-202.

75.   Sarasua, S. and D.A. Savitz, *Cured and broiled meat consumption in relation to childhood cancer: Denver, Colorado (United States).* Cancer Causes Control, 1994. **5**(2): p. 141-8.

76.   Bunin, G.R., et al., *Maternal diet and risk of astrocytic glioma in children: a report from the Childrens Cancer Group (United States and Canada).* Cancer Causes Control, 1994. **5**(2): p. 177-87.

77.   Medicine, P.C.f.R. *Fecal Contamination in Retail Chicken Products: A Report from the Physicians Committee for Responsible Medicine April 2012.* 2012 [cited 2013 February 26, 2013]; Available from: http://www.pcrm.org/health/reports/fecal-contamination-in-retail-chicken-products.

78.   He, K., et al., *Accumulated evidence on fish consumption and coronary heart disease mortality: a meta-analysis of cohort studies.* Circulation, 2004. **109**(22): p. 2705-11.

79.   *<What You Need to Know About Mercury in Fish and Shellfish.pdf>.*

80.   PETA. *PETA Offers $1 Million Reward to First to Make In Vitro Meat.* 2013 February 19, 2013]; Available from: http://www.peta.org/features/In-Vitro-Meat-Contest.aspx.

81.   Jacobson, M.F., *Adverse reactions linked to Quorn-brand foods.* Allergy, 2003. **58**(5): p. 455-456.

82.   Barnard, N. *Dr. Neal Barnard On Why Milk is Harmful | The Kind Life*. The Kind Life 2013 1/8/2013 [cited 2015 March 12, 2015]; Available from: http://thekindlife.com/blog/2013/01/why-milk-is-harmful-by-dr-neal-barnard/.

83.   Feskanich, D., W.C. Willett, and G.A. Colditz, *Calcium, vitamin D, milk consumption, and hip fractures: a prospective study among postmenopausal women.* Am J Clin Nutr, 2003. **77**(2): p. 504-11.

84.   Lanou, A.J., S.E. Berkow, and N.D. Barnard, *Calcium, dairy products, and bone health in children and young adults: a reevaluation of the evidence.* Pediatrics, 2005. **115**(3): p. 736-43.

85.   Sonneville, K.R., et al., *Vitamin d, calcium, and dairy intakes and stress fractures among female adolescents.* Arch Pediatr Adolesc Med, 2012. **166**(7): p. 595-600.

86.   Lanou, A.J. and N.D. Barnard, *Dairy and weight loss hypothesis: an evaluation of the clinical trials.* Nutr Rev, 2008. **66**(5): p. 272-279.

87.   Berkey, C.S., et al., *Milk, dairy fat, dietary calcium, and weight gain: a longitudinal study of adolescents.* Arch Pediatr Adolesc Med,

2005. **159**(6): p. 543-50.

88.   Lanou, A.J., *Data do not support recommending dairy products for weight loss.* Obes Res, 2005. **13**(1): p. 191.

89.   In his book, M., the deadly poison, Robert Cohen.

90.   Engdahl, F.W., *Seeds of Destruction: The Hidden Agenda of Genetic Manipulation.* 2007, Montreal, Quebec: Global Research.

91.   Hankinson, S.E., et al., *Circulating concentrations of insulin-like growth factor-I and risk of breast cancer.* Lancet, 1998. **351**(9113): p. 1393-6.

92.   Yu, H. and T. Rohan, *Role of the insulin-like growth factor family in cancer development and progression.* J Natl Cancer Inst, 2000. **92**(18): p. 1472-89.

93.   Pan, S.Y., et al., *A case-control study of diet and the risk of ovarian cancer.* Cancer Epidemiol Biomarkers Prev, 2004. **13**(9): p. 1521-7.

94.   Kimura, T., et al., *Gastrointestinal absorption of recombinant human insulin-like growth factor-I in rats.* J Pharmacol Exp Ther, 1997. **283**(2): p. 611-8.

95.   Biro, F.M., et al., *Pubertal Assessment Method and Baseline Characteristics in a Mixed Longitudinal Study of Girls.* Pediatrics, 2010.

96.   Divall, S.A., et al., *Divergent roles of growth factors in the GnRH regulation of puberty in mice.* J Clin Invest, 2010. **120**(8): p. 2900-9.

97.   Wiley, A.S., *Milk intake and total dairy consumption: associations with early menarche in NHANES 1999-2004.* PLoS One, 2011. **6**(2): p. 0014685.

98.   Ramezani Tehrani, F., et al., *Intake of dairy products, calcium, magnesium, and phosphorus in childhood and age at menarche in the tehran lipid and glucose study.* PLoS One, 2013. **8**(2): p. 25.

99.   Adebamowo, C.A., et al., *High school dietary dairy intake and teenage acne.* J Am Acad Dermatol, 2005. **52**(2): p. 207-214.

100.   Adebamowo, C.A., et al., *Milk consumption and acne in adolescent girls.* Dermatol Online J, 2006. **12**(4): p. 1.

101.   Melnik, B.C., *Evidence for acne-promoting effects of milk and other insulinotropic dairy products.* Nestle Nutr Workshop Ser Pediatr Program, 2011. **67**: p. 131-45.

102.   *Lactose Intolerance | Johns Hopkins Medicine Health Library.* 2015; Available from: http://www.hopkinsmedicine.org/healthlibrary/conditions/digestiv e_disorders/lactose_intolerance_85,P00388/.

103.   Brannon, P.M., et al., *NIH Consensus Development Conference*

Statement: Lactose Intolerance and Health. NIH Consens State Sci Statements, 2010. **27**(2).

104. Park, M., et al., *Consumption of milk and calcium in midlife and the future risk of Parkinson disease.* Neurology, 2005. **64**(6): p. 1047-51.

105. Abbott, R.D., et al., *Midlife milk consumption and substantia nigra neuron density at death.* Neurology, 2016. **86**(6): p. 512-9.

106. Macdonald, L.E., et al., *A systematic review and meta-analysis of the effects of pasteurization on milk vitamins, and evidence for raw milk consumption and other health-related outcomes.* J Food Prot, 2011. **74**(11): p. 1814-32.

107. Klaper, M. 1985.

108. Cook, M.S. *Harvard Declares Dairy NOT Part of Healthy Diet.* 2012.

109. Concerns, U.P., *<Free-Range Poulry and Eggs.pdf>.*

110. Jacob, J.a.R.M. *<Designer and Specialty Eggs.pdf>.* 2012.

111. Freese, W. and D. Schubert, *Safety testing and regulation of genetically engineered foods.* Biotechnol Genet Eng Rev, 2004. **21**: p. 299-324.

112. Group, E., *Putting the Cartel before the Horse ... and Farm, Seeds, Soil, Peasants, etc. .* 2013.

113. Smith, J.M., *Seeds of Deception: Exposing Industry and Government Lies About the Safety of the Genetically Engineered Foods* 2003, Fairfield, Iowa: Yes! Books.

114. Robin, M.-M., *The World According to Monsanto: Pollution, Corruption, and the Control of our Food Supply.* 2008, New York: The New Press.

115. Lotter, D., *Genetic Engineering and the Failure of Science - Part 2: Academic Capitalism and the Loss of Scientific Integrity.pdf.* International Journal of Sociology of Agriculture and Food, 2009. **Volume 16**(issue 1 (2009)): p. 50-68.

116. Responsibility, E.N.o.S.f.S.a.E. *ENSSER Statement, 21 October 2013.* 2013 October 21, 2013 [Available from: http://sustainablepulse.com/wp-content/uploads/ENSSER Statement no scientific consensus on GMO safety ENG LV.pdf.

117. Gurian-Sherman, D., *Failure to Yield: Evaluating the Performance of Genetically Engineered Crops.* 2009, Union of Concerned Scientists

118. Heinemann, J.A., et al., *Sustainability and innovation in staple crop production in the US Midwest.* International Journal of Agricultural Sustainability, 2013: p. 1-18.

119. Shi, G., J.P. Chavas, and J. Lauer, *Commercialized transgenic traits,*

maize productivity and yield risk. Nat Biotechnol, 2013. **31**(2): p. 111-4.

120. *Water Pollution Facts.* 2014.
121. Capel, P., *Widely Used Herbicide Commonly Found in Rain and Streams in the Mississippi River Basin.* 2011, U.S. Department of the Interior, U.S. Geological Survey.
122. Scientists, U.o.C., *High and Dry: Why Genetic Engineering is Not Solving Agriculture's Drought Problem in a Thirsty World.* 2012.
123. Repository, F.A.O.C.D., *What is Agrobiodiversity?... PDF version.*
124. Vadakattu, G., and Watson, S., *<Ecologial Impaks of GM Cotton on Soil Biodiversity.pdf>.* 2004.
125. Shiva, V., *Monsanto and the Seeds of Suicide.* 2014.
126. Gilbert, S., *Monsanto's Ever-Stronger Stranglehold on the Seed Industry - DailyFinance.* 2014.
127. Senauer, B. *The Appetite for Biofuel Starves the Poor.* 2008.
128. Wise, J., *Forget Overcrowding. The World Population Could Start Declining.* 2014.
129. Pimentel, D., *Impacts of Organic Farming on the Efficiency of Energy Use in Agriculture*, in *An Organic Center State of Science Review*, T.O. Center, Editor. 2006, Cornell University: Itaca, NY.
130. *Can Organic Farming Feed Us All? | Worldwatch Institute. 2014.* **2014**.
131. Kopicki, A., *Strong Support for Labeling Modified Foods*, in *The New York Times.* 2013, The New York Times.
132. Muir, P., *III. ARE PEST LOSSES DECREASING?* 2013. **2013**.
133. Miller, G.T., *Sustaining the Earth.* 6th ed. 2004, Pacific Grove, California: Thomson Learning, Inc.
134. Weisskopf, M.G., et al., *Persistent organochlorine pesticides in serum and risk of Parkinson disease.* Neurology, 2010. **74**(13): p. 1055-61.
135. Boyle, C.A., et al., *Trends in the prevalence of developmental disabilities in US children, 1997-2008.* Pediatrics, 2011. **127**(6): p. 1034-42.
136. Shelton, J.F., I. Hertz-Picciotto, and I.N. Pessah, *Tipping the balance of autism risk: potential mechanisms linking pesticides and autism.* Environ Health Perspect, 2012. **120**(7): p. 944-51.
137. Hertz-Picciotto, I. and L. Delwiche, *The rise in autism and the role of age at diagnosis.* Epidemiology, 2009. **20**(1): p. 84-90.
138. Kristin S. Schafer, K.S., Marquez, Emily C., *A Generation in Jeopardy: How Pesticides Are Undermining Our Children's Health &*

Intelligence. 2012, Pesticide Action Network.

139. Richard, S., et al., *Differential Effects of Glyphosate and Roundup on Human Placental Cells and Aromatase.* Environmental Health Perspectives, 2005. **113**(6): p. 716-720.

140. Benachour, N. and G.E. Seralini, *Glyphosate formulations induce apoptosis and necrosis in human umbilical, embryonic, and placental cells.* Chem Res Toxicol, 2009. **22**(1): p. 97-105.

141. Vogt, R., et al., *Cancer and non-cancer health effects from food contaminant exposures for children and adults in California: a risk assessment.* Environmental Health, 2012. **11**(1): p. 83.

142. Thongprakaisang, S., et al., *Glyphosate induces human breast cancer cells growth via estrogen receptors.* Food and Chemical Toxicology, 2013. **59**(0): p. 129-136.

143. Taetzsch, T. and M.L. Block, *Pesticides, microglial NOX2, and Parkinson's disease.* J Biochem Mol Toxicol, 2013. **27**(2): p. 137-49.

144. Wang, A., et al., *Parkinson's disease risk from ambient exposure to pesticides.* Eur J Epidemiol, 2011. **26**(7): p. 547-55.

145. *<Pesticides and Reproductive Harm.pdf>*.

146. Wei, Y., J. Zhu, and A. Nguyen, *Urinary concentrations of dichlorophenol pesticides and obesity among adult participants in the U.S. National Health and Nutrition Examination Survey (NHANES) 2005-2008.* Int J Hyg Environ Health, 2013.

147. Casals-Casas, C. and B. Desvergne, *Endocrine disruptors: from endocrine to metabolic disruption.* Annu Rev Physiol, 2011. **73**: p. 135-62.

148. Valvi, D., et al., *Prenatal concentrations of polychlorinated biphenyls, DDE, and DDT and overweight in children: a prospective birth cohort study.* Environ Health Perspect, 2012. **120**(3): p. 451-7.

149. Barrett, J.R., *OP Pesticides in Children's Bodies: The Effects of a Conventional versus Organic Diet.* Environmental Health Perspectives, 2006. **114**(2): p. A112-A112.

150. Baranski, M., et al., *Higher antioxidant and lower cadmium concentrations and lower incidence of pesticide residues in organically grown crops: a systematic literature review and meta-analyses.* Br J Nutr, 2014. **112**(5): p. 794-811.

151. Curl, C.L., et al., *Estimating Pesticide Exposure from Dietary Intake and Organic Food Choices: The Multi-Ethnic Study of Atherosclerosis (MESA).* Environ Health Perspect, 2015.

152. Guyenet, S. *By 2606, the US Diet will be 100 Percent Sugar.* Whole Health Source 2012; Available from:

http://wholehealthsource.blogspot.com/2012/02/by-2606-us-diet-will-be-100-percent.html.

153. Basu, S., et al., *The relationship of sugar to population-level diabetes prevalence: an econometric analysis of repeated cross-sectional data.* PLoS One, 2013. **8**(2): p. e57873.

154. Hyman, M., *Eggs Don't Cause Heart Attacks -- Sugar Does*, in *Huffpost Healthy Living*. 2014.

155. Lenoir, M., et al., *Intense sweetness surpasses cocaine reward.* PLoS One, 2007. **2**(8): p. e698.

156. Avena, N.M., P. Rada, and B.G. Hoebel, *Evidence for sugar addiction: behavioral and neurochemical effects of intermittent, excessive sugar intake.* Neurosci Biobehav Rev, 2008. **32**(1): p. 20-39.

157. Burger, K.S. and E. Stice, *Variability in reward responsivity and obesity: evidence from brain imaging studies.* Curr Drug Abuse Rev, 2011. **4**(3): p. 182-9.

158. Stice, E., et al., *The contribution of brain reward circuits to the obesity epidemic.* Neurosci Biobehav Rev, 2013. **37**(9 Pt A): p. 2047-58.

159. Parker, H., *Princeton University - A sweet problem: Princeton researchers find that high-fructose corn syrup prompts considerably more weight gain.* News at Princeton, 2014.

160. Trocho, C., et al., *Formaldehyde derived from dietary aspartame binds to tissue components in vivo.* Life Sci, 1998. **63**(5): p. 337-49.

161. Schernhammer, E.S., et al., *Consumption of artificial sweetener- and sugar-containing soda and risk of lymphoma and leukemia in men and women.* Am J Clin Nutr, 2012. **96**(6): p. 1419-28.

162. Zhang, G.H., et al., *Effects of mother's dietary exposure to acesulfame-K in Pregnancy or lactation on the adult offspring's sweet preference.* Chem Senses, 2011. **36**(9): p. 763-70.

163. Price, J.M., et al., *Bladder tumors in rats fed cyclohexylamine or high doses of a mixture of cyclamate and saccharin.* Science, 1970. **167**(3921): p. 1131-2.

164. Schiffman, S.S. and K.I. Rother, *Sucralose, a synthetic organochlorine sweetener: overview of biological issues.* J Toxicol Environ Health B Crit Rev, 2013. **16**(7): p. 399-451.

165. Dong, S., et al., *Polychlorinated dibenzo-p-dioxins and dibenzofurans formed from sucralose at high temperatures.* Scientific Reports, 2013. **3**: p. 2946.

166. Kobylewski, S., Eckhert, Curtis D. Ph.d., *Toxicology of Rebaudioside A.: A Review*. 2008, Department of Environmental Health and

Sciences, Molecular Technology UCLA School of Public Health Los Angeles, California.

167.   Fowler, S.P., et al., *Fueling the obesity epidemic? Artificially sweetened beverage use and long-term weight gain.* Obesity (Silver Spring), 2008. **16**(8): p. 1894-900.

168.   Stellman, S.D. and L. Garfinkel, *Artificial sweetener use and one-year weight change among women.* Prev Med, 1986. **15**(2): p. 195-202.

169.   Swithers, S.E., C.R. Baker, and T.L. Davidson, *General and persistent effects of high-intensity sweeteners on body weight gain and caloric compensation in rats.* Behav Neurosci, 2009. **123**(4): p. 772-80.

170.   Mancino, L. and F. Kuchler, *Demand for whole-grain bread before and after the release of Dietary Guidelines.* Applied Economic Perspectives and Policy, 2011.

171.   Davis, W., *Wheat Belly: Lose the Wheat, Lose the Weight, and Find Your Path Back to Health.* 2011, New York: Rodale.

172.   Smyth, D.J., et al., *Shared and distinct genetic variants in type 1 diabetes and celiac disease.* N Engl J Med, 2008. **359**(26): p. 2767-77.

173.   Institute, T.C. *Prominent Government Watchdog Asks Obama Administration to Remove Organic Leadership at USDA.* 2015 April 24, 2015 [cited 2015; Available from: http://www.cornucopia.org/2015/04/prominent-government-watchdog-asks-obama-administration-to-remove-organic-leadership-at-usda/.

174.   Cohen, J.F.W., et al., *Impact of the New U.S. Department of Agriculture School Meal Standards on Food Selection, Consumption, and Waste.* American Journal of Preventive Medicine. **46**(4): p. 388-394.

175.   Weinstein, M., *The Surprising Power of Family Meals: How Eating Together Makes Us Smarter, Stronger, Healthier, and Happier.* 2005, Hanover, N.H.: Steerforth Press.

176.   Abuse, T.N.C.o.A.a.S., *The Importance of FamilyDinners VIII*, in *The Importance of Family Dinners*. 2012, Columbia Univrsity.

Index

2,5-dichlorophenol, 194
Acesulfame K, 213
Acesulfame potassium, 213
acne, 154
ADHD, 96, 191
ALA (alinolenic acid), 110
allergies, 26, 115, 155, 156, 224
alloxan, 221
alpha-linolenic acid, 164
Alzheimer's, 26, 190
American Academy of
   Pediatricians, 127
American Cancer Society, 51, 152,
   218
American Dairy Association, 157
American Diabetes Association,
   205
American Heart Association, 25,
   51, 60, 102, 207, 234
American Humane Certified, 163
*American Journal of Clinical
   Nutrition*, 106
American Medical Association,
   127
American Nurses Association,
   127, 152
American Public Health
   Association,, 126, 152
American Society for the
   Prevention of Cruelty to
   Animals
   SPCA, 134
Animal Welfare Approved, 163
antibiotics, 72, 126, 127, 133,
   134, 137, 138, 139, 145, 151,
153, 156, 161, 162, 163, 205,
   229, 230
Aqua Bounty Farms, 141, 182
arsenic, 187, 192
arteriolosclerosis, 25
aspartame, 183, 212, 213, 215,
   216, 217, 220, 246
asthma, 23, 26, 86, 91, 96, 99,
   154, 156, 190, 195, 241
atrazine, 195
autism, 26, 190, 191
azodicarbonamide, 83, 86, 87,
   248
Barnard, Dr. Neal D., 148
battery-cage poultry production,
   163
beta-adrenoceptor agonists, 128
Betty Crocker, 47, 95
Beyond Pesticides, 192, 196, 201
BHA, 70, 87, 93, 246
BHT, 70, 88, 93, 246
birth defects, 55, 93, 162, 190,
   191, 195
bisphenol A, 54, 55, 251, *See* BPA
black hole tactics, 44
boric acid, 198
BPA, 54, 55, 56, 57, 58, 60, 251
Breast Cancer Fund, 56
Brownell, Kelly, 78
bST
   bovine somatotropin. *See*
      bovine growth hormone
cage free, 138, 163
calcium propionate, 83, 88, 246
Campbell's, 47, 56, 57

cancer, 21, 23, 25, 55, 82, 84, 86, 87, 88, 89, 93, 101, 104, 108, 109, 121, 129, 130, 134, 135, 136, 152, 154, 156, 157, 159, 188, 190, 192, 193, 197, 207, 213, 214, 217, 242

cardiovascular disease, 25, 56, 102, 106, 109, 113, 204

Carrageenan, 88

Carson, Rachel, 189

Castelli, William, 105

caveat emptor, 46

CDC, 21, 22, 24, 56, 57, 77, 90

celiac disease, 26, 132, 222, 223, 224, 225, 226, 227

Celiac Disease Foundation, 224, 227

cellulose, 69, 88, 133, 247

Center for Behavioral Medicine, 212

Center for Food Safety, 152

Center for Science in the Public Interest, 69, 93, 95, 96, 121, 126, 143

Certified Humane, 52, 134, 163

Channel One, 34

Chili's, 166

Chipotle, 145, 158

chlordane, 192

Christopher Columbus, 203

chronic bronchitis, 23

Citrus Red, 94

Coca-Cola, 32, 181

cochineal, 98

cochineal extract, 98

Codex Alimentarius, 71

colitis, 26, 89

community supported agriculture programs (CSAs), 185

ConAgra, 52, 71, 90

ConAgra Foods, 52

Confined Animal Feeding Operations, (CAFOs), 133

Confined Feeding Operations (CAFOs), 229

Consumers Union, 134, 198

Country of Origin Labeling (COOL), 53

Crohn's disease, 26

CSPI, 67, 70, 74, 122, 131, 142, 143, 213, 214, 216

CSPI (Center for Science in the Public Interest), 50

Daily Finance, 176

Dannon, 161

DARK Act, 182, 183

DARK Act., 183

Davis, Dr. William, 223

DDE, 188, 192, 194, 199

DDT, 187, 188, 189, 191, 192, 194, 199

DEHP, 54, 57, 60

Delaney Clause, 84

Dermatitis Herpetiformis Duhring's Disease, 224

DHA (docosahexaenoic acid), 109

Diacetyl, 90

dieldrin, 193

Dieldrin, 192

dioxin, 192

disodium guanylate, 91

diverticulitis, 26

Dow, 168, 181

Dr. Ralph G. Walton, Dr. Ralph G., 212

DRIs
  Dietary Reference Intakes, 62

DroughtGard, 173

DRVs
  Daily Reference Value, 62

Duhring's disease, 224
E coli, 131
early puberty, 153, 154, 193, 195
Enig, Dr. Mary G., 104
enriched, 64, 66, 221, 226
EPA, 109, 110, 139, 140, 191, 192, 196, 198, 201, 241
EPA (eicosapentaenoic acid), 109
Epstein, Dr. Samuel S., 130
Equal, 211
estradiol, 129
estrogen, 55, 56, 93, 159
Estrogen, 129
European Union, 56, 87, 90, 97, 128, 129, 138, 151, 180
Fair Trade label, 52
Fallon, Sally, 104
FDA, 45, 47, 48, 49, 50, 56, 57, 59, 62, 63, 65, 66, 67, 68, 69, 70, 71, 74, 77, 78, 84, 85, 86, 87, 89, 90, 91, 92, 93, 94, 96, 111, 115, 118, 120, 121, 122, 126, 128, 129, 130, 131, 134, 138, 139, 150, 151, 156, 157, 161, 163, 167, 182, 211, 213, 214, 215, 216, 217, 225, 236, 241, 242
Feingold, Dr. Benjamin, 95
folic acid, 64, 66, 226, 247
Food Additives Amendment, 84, 85
Food Allergen Labeling and Consumer Protection Act of 2004, 118
Food and Agriculture Organization of the United Nations, 71
Food Animal Concerns Trust (FACT), 126

Food Safety Modernization Act, 156
Food, Drug, and Cosmetic Act, 118
fortified, 64, 66, 79, 159, 221, 252
FPLA
    Fair Packaging and Labeling Act, 45
Framingham Study, 105
    Framingham Heart Study, 105
free range, 138, 163, 164
Friedman, Dr. Jeffrey, 206
Frito-lay, 98
Frito-Lay, 71
Froot Loops, 52
General Mills, 29, 52, 69, 95, 181, 236
generally recognized as safe, 85, 89
genistein, 193
Gilbert, Sarah, 176
Gluten Sensitivity, 224
Glyphosate, 172, 193
glysophate, 120, 173, 192
GMO labeling initiatives, 38, 230
GMOs, 71, 173, 175, 177, 179, 180, 183, 185, 230
Gossypol, 116
GRAS
    generally recognized as safe, 85, 88, 89, 90, 91, 115, 167, 211, 216, 217
Great for You, 77
Greenpeace, 178
Grocery Manufacturers Association, 67, 181, 236
Guiding Stars, 76
Guyenet, Dr. Stephen, 204
H.112, 181
halo effect, 60

halo\ effect, 53
Harvard Nurses' Health Study, 148
Harvard School of Public Health, 66, 75, 121, 157, 191, 197
Health and Human Services (HHS, 75
health claims, 36, 49, 50, 61
HFCS
  High Fructose Corn Syrup, 210
Hoebel, Bart, 210
Hoebel, Dr. Bart, 208
Hunt, Patricia, 55
Hyman, Dr. Mark, 207
hyper palatable foods, 36
hyper-vitaminosis, 66
IGF-1, 150, 152, 153, 156
Irritable Bowel syndrome (IBS), 89
Irritable Bowel Syndrome (IBS), 26
ischemic heart disease, 24
isoflavone, 159
Kellogg, 29, 52, 71, 74, 95
Keys, Ancel, 102
kidney disease, 23
Klaper, Dr. Michael, 157
Klum, Heidi, 51
Kraft, 161
Kroger, 158
Lactobacilli, 160
lactose intolerance, 157
Lactose intolerance, 155
lauric acid, 115, 159
learning disabilities, 190, 195
leptin resistance, 206, 207
leukemia, 25, 87, 136
Lipid Hypothesis, 102
Lou Gehrig, 51
Lustig, Dr. Robert, 207
lutein, 162

macular degeneration (AMD), 162
Mad Cow, 115
maltodextrin, 69, 131
Marketplace Surveillance Program of the California Department of Pesticide Regulation, 198
McDonald's, 32, 33, 131
meat glue, 132
Meat Inspection Act of 1906, 83
mechanically deboned meats (MDM, 131
Metabolic Syndrome, 24
methylene chloride, 213
Milwaukee Journal Sentinel, 55
monolaurin, 159
monosodium glutamate. *See* MSG
Monsanto, 120, 150, 151, 152, 167, 168, 171, 172, 173, 174, 175, 180, 181
MSG, 85, 88, 91, 92, 99, 132, 247, 249
Muir, Dr. Patricia, 190
Müller, Paul Hermann, 187
multiple sclerosis (MS), 224
My Pyramid, 75
mycoprotein, 142, 143
MyPlate, 31, 32, 75, 76
Nabisco., 121
Nancy's All Natural, 161
National Dairy Council, 149
National Institute for Occupational Safety and Health (OSHA), 90
National Institute on Drug Abuse, 208
National Toxicology Program (NTP), 55, 214
NatraTaste, 211
neonicotinoids, 195

Neotame, 211, 215, 216
NesQuik, 42
Nestlé, 42
Nestle, Marion, 50, 51, 120
Niacin, 138
NIH
    National Intitute of Health, 155
nitrite, 85, 136, 137, 145, 246
NLEA. *See* Nutrition Standards
    Alphabet
Non-GMO Project, 181, 184
Non-GMO Project Verified, 181
NutraSweet, 211
Nutrition Facts panel, 61
Nutrition Facts Panel, 46, 59, 61,
    64, 69, 70, 74
Nutrition Journal, 134
Nutrition Keys, 77
Nutrition Labeling and Education
    Act, 36, 61
Nuval, 76
Obama, Michelle, 77, 233
Olestra, 120, 121, 123, 247
Oliver, Jamie, 131, 132, 235
Omega-3, 65, 109, 110, 115, 117,
    119, 122, 164, 166
Omega-6, 115, 116, 117, 118,
    119, 122
Oregon Research Institute, 208
osteoporosis, 148, 224
Outback Steakhouse, 166
P.F. Chang's, 166
PAMTA
    The Preservation of Antibiotics
        for Medical Treatment Act,
        127
paraquat, 193
Parkinson's, 190, 193
pasteurization, 156
PCBs, 139, 140, 194

penicillin, 126
People for the Ethical Treatment
    of Animals (PETA, 142
PepsiCo, 29, 52, 87, 216
Pesticide Data Program of the
    U.S. Department of Agriculture,
    198
pesticides, 70, 72, 73, 85, 134,
    137, 138, 161, 162, 171, 172,
    175, 176, 179, 184, 187, 188,
    189, 190, 191, 192, 193, 194,
    195, 196, 198, 200, 201, 229,
    261
phthalates, 57, 60
Physicians Committee for
    Responsible Medicine, 148
Physicians for Responsible
    Medicine, 138, 235
phytoestrogen, 159, 193
pink slime, 131
Pizza Hut, 35
PKU
    phenylketonuria, 212
Plastic Coding, 58, 250
PLU # (price look up) sticker, 184
plumping, 133
Pollan, Michael, 104, 143
polydextrose, 69, 247
Popcorn Worker's Lung, 90
Post, 29
potassium bromate, 83, 92, 93,
    100
Potassium bromate, 92
precocious puberty, 129, 153
Price, Dr. Weston, 104, 115
Prior-sanctioned substances, 85
probiotics, 65
progesterone,, 129
Prop 52, 38
Prop. 37, 38

Propyl gallate, 93
Publix Super Markets, 158
Quorn-brand frozen meat
   substitute, 142
ractopamine, 128, 129, 145
Ravnskov, Uffe, 104
rBGH, 145, 150, 151, 152, 153,
   158, 161, 165
   bovine growth hormone, 150
RDAs
   Recommended Daily
      Allowances, 62
Recommended Dietary
   Allowances, 144
Red Dye No. 4, 94
rhinitis, 154
Rodale Institute's Farming
   Systems Trial, 179
Rosa Mexicano, 166
rotenone, 193
Roundup, 171, 172, 182, 192
Rudd Center for Food Policy and
   Obesity, 33, 78, 218
Saccharin, 211, 213
Safeway, 77, 158
Safeway Dairy Group, 158
salatrim, 122
salmonella, 131
Sam's Club, 158
Schlossser, Eric, 143
Seafood Safe, 140
Selenium, 62, 138
self-endorsement labeling
   systems, 52
Shiva, Vandana, 176
significant scientific agreement
   (SSA), 48
SimpleNutrition, 77
slack fill, 43, 45, 59
Smart Choices, 52

sodium nitrate, 135, 137
sodium nitrites, 137
sodium stearoyl lactate, 83
soy, 31, 73, 108, 113, 114, 116,
   129, 141, 142, 156, 159, 160,
   180, 184, 233, 247
Splenda, 75, 214, 215
Spock, Dr. Benjamin, 148
Stallone, Sylvester, 51
Stampfer, Dr. Meir, 121
Standard American Diet (SAD), 26
statement of identity, 47, 161
Stice, Eric, 208
Structure/function claims, 50
sulfites, 93
Sulfites, 93
Surgeon General, 23
Taco Bell, 35
Taylor, Michael R., 151
testosterone, 57, 129
tetracycline, 126
TG enzyme
   TGP enzyme, 132
The American Medical
   Association, 102
The British Medical Journal, 118
The Cancer Prevention Coalition,
   152
The Cornucopia Institute, 89
The Institute of Medicine (IOM),
   77
The International Food Additives
   Council, 82
*The Journal of Child and
   Adolescent Health*, 96
*The Journal of Consumer
   Research*, 47
*The Journal of the American
   Medical Association*, 106
The Lancet, 87, 96

The National Institute of Health, 105, 113

The Women's Health Initiative Dietary Modification Trial,, 106

Tobacman, Dr. Joanne, 89

tocopherols, 118

tocotrienols, 118

Trader Joes, 100

Trans fats, 48, 63, 69, 110, 111, 112, 115, 116, 118, 120, 122, 161

transglutaminase, 132

Twinkies, 31, 47

Type 2 diabetes, 21, 24, 56, 103, 194, 205, 207

Tyson Foods, 52

U.N. Food and Agriculture Organization (FAO), 30

U.S. Department of Agriculture (USDA), 31

U.S. Government Accountability Office (GAO), 50

U.S. PIRG, 31

Union of Concerned Scientists, 126, 134, 170

United Nations Food Safety Agency, 151

United Poultry Concerns, 163

University of Arkansas Division of Agriculture,, 137

University of California Davis, 192

USDA
  United States Department of Agriculture, 31, 71, 72, 73, 75, 80, 85, 130, 133, 134, 135, 138, 140, 156, 157, 158, 163, 168, 171, 173, 184, 195, 199, 213, 219, 225, 229, 230, 231, 233

Vitamin E, 119, 136, 246

Volk, Marion, 104

Volkow, Dr. Nora, 208

Wal-Mart, 77, 158

Wesson Oil, 71

Wheat allergy, 225

Wheeler-Lea Act, 84

WHO
  World Health Organization, 25, 86

Whole Foods, 100, 145

Wiley, Dr. Harvey W., 84

Women, Infants and Children (WIC) program, 21

World Health Organization, 25, 86, 87, 93, 127

World Trade Organization, 53, 130

Yale University, 33, 52

Yellow dye #5, 96

Yoplait, 161

zeaxanthin, 162

CPSIA information can be obtained at www.ICGtesting.com
Printed in the USA
LVOW10s1803221016

509860LV00011B/55/P